Praise for W

Inspirational, enlight *bridges the gap between integrative and conventional medicine and supports your journey to healing. I highly recommend it.*

– Dr. Anna Cabeca, DO, OBGYN, FACOG, bestselling author of The Hormone Fix, Keto-Green 16 and MenuPause

Gary Kaplan is not only a pioneer in his field, he's a badass who is changing the face of medicine. This book holds everything I wish I knew twenty years ago about autoimmunity. It's an incredible resource for anyone with chronic pain and illness. It will bring hope and health to so many people.

– Dave Asprey, founder, Bulletproof 360

"What am I missing? What do others like me know that I don't? I think there must be an answer out there for my pain and suffering what with all the fantastic medical advances of the last few years. I just don't know what it is and sometimes I feel despair." If these thoughts have been going through your mind, then this book is for you. It provides a path and plan to finally alleviate your pain and suffering and return you to a time when you could just be you. This book is a breakthrough and a revelation and can truly help where others have failed.

– Richard Rossi

When patients get told for the fifth time that their symptoms are all in their head, a window should open and Dr. Kaplan's book should come sailing though. This is critical book should be read by every medical student, nurse, and physician.

– Sarah Ramey
Author of the critically acclaimed book
The Lady's Handbook for her Mysterious Illness

Dr. Kaplan takes us on a journey of understanding our immune mechanisms and the havoc that can occur when a system designed to protect from infection turns against us, resulting in autoimmunity. With the creative use of analogies, such as the "ravaging raccoons," he helps us understand that a heightened immune response directed at our own cells can create a diverse constellation of symptoms from chronic fatigue to depression, irritable bowel and POTS. Touching vignettes from his own patients' experiences illustrate the pitfalls of just treating individual symptoms and the critical need to identify and treat the underlying infectious disease at the root of the problem. Dr. Kaplan's compassionate approach brings striking clarity to overwhelming symptoms and provides patients with a roadmap to recovery.

**– Helene A. Emsellem, MD, Director,
The Center for Sleep & Wake Disorders**

Our current healthcare system and research capability has mostly failed to help our patients with chronic, complex, and costly autoimmune diseases. Patients with these conditions feel lost and dismissed in our healthcare system. They have learned they need to educate themselves in order to navigate through the confusion and be better advocates for effective healthcare. Our immune system protects us, but past infections and chronic, difficult to detect current infections and other danger triggers can provoke our immune system to cause chronic illness. The Step-By-Step Guide to Recovery section of the book helps patients to understand treatment options that are available. Knowledge of these options helps patients make better informed consent decisions. In short, Dr Kaplan's book gives the general public knowledge of both complex autoimmune disease and treatment options; and knowledge is empowering.

**– Robert C Bransfield, MD, Distinguished Life Fellow,
American Psychiatric Association**

WHY YOU ARE STILL SICK

Infections that Trigger Autoimmunity
&
What You Can Do About It

GARY KAPLAN, DO
DONNA BEECH

Callanan Publishers
Washington, D.C.

First paperback edition June 2022

Book design by Mr. Wolf

ISBN 978-0-578-39394-0 (paperback)

www.kaplanclinic.com

WHY YOU ARE STILL SICK

*To Fran, my best friend, my wife,
who blesses me with her love, support,
wisdom and faith in me.*

TABLE OF CONTENTS

PART I

DO YOU HAVE AUTOIMMUNE DISEASE?

.

CHAPTER 1
—
MISSED INFECTIONS

Autoimmune disease creeps up on you. It starts with the aches and pains. At first you dismiss them with a shrug. You tell yourself you had a hard day. You shouldn't have lifted that big box. You're not getting any younger. But the time between new aches and pains keeps getting shorter. Your ability to bounce back starts to wane. You catch the flu, and it takes weeks instead of days to recover. Before you know it, something is always tweaked or hurting. It's harder to do things you used to do with ease. You keep adapting, trying to adjust, accommodating each new pain and limitation, until one day you hardly recognize yourself.

Whether you notice it or not, your life is getting smaller. You don't have the interest or the energy to pursue the things you used to enjoy. Things you used to take in stride now keep you up at night feeling anxious. Low-grade depression hovers over you like a cloud.

What's worse is the pills aren't helping. You've gone to the doctor and tried medication for anxiety or depression. It helped at first, but then, as if you'd slid down a muddy embankment, you found yourself right back where you started. Nothing you do seems to work for long. Antacids aren't improving your digestion. Sleeping pills can't keep you asleep. So, you stare at the ceiling in the dark, wondering what's gone wrong.

One day soon a new symptom will introduce itself. Maybe you haven't reached this moment yet, but if things keep going as they are, you will. Sometimes it starts with a sharp inexplicable pain in your hip or a migraine like you've never had before. Whether your doctor recognizes it or not, it's a tipping point. This is not just one more pain; it's a sign that things have gone too far. Your immune system is completely overloaded, and your symptoms have started to cascade. You may look fine, but you are really very sick. You've crossed the line into *autoimmune disease*.

When immunologists use the word *immunity*, they are describing the immune system's appropriate response to a pathogen. Antibodies have been produced. Defensive cells have been released to fight off an attacker.[1] To have *autoimmunity* (literally, *immunity to one's self*) means that your immune system has turned that same immune response against you.

With an autoimmune disease, your immune system has gotten confused about what in your body is friend or foe. Instead of attacking bacterial invaders and infections, it attacks your own healthy tissue. This is nothing to take lightly. It is a failure of your body's fundamental defense system. It means something has gone terribly wrong.

It's an urgent problem, but one that is still, unfortunately, very difficult to diagnose. Once your symptoms start cascading, multiple organs are affected. As soon as your doctor treats one set of symptoms, another will appear. Since the trouble is with the immune system, its dysfunction can affect any system in the body. Fix the hip pain and it can show up as a migraine. Fix your sleep and your digestion may get worse. The underlying problem is completely unaffected by tamping down the symptoms. So, it looks as if it's just moving around, but in fact, the real problem is never being treated at all.

As you can imagine, any conventional doctor will start to wonder what's going on when they treat your headache and you say, "But now my back hurts!" Most doctors aren't taught that when symptoms move around, it may well be a sign of systemic inflammation. It's far more common for them to see patients who suffer from anxiety about symptoms that they've read about online. If someone keeps returning with new complaints, they're likely to assume it's psychological.

Autoimmune disease is a condition of pathological inflammation. Autoimmune disease does not always attack the nervous system, but when it does, it produces symptoms that ebb and flare like a forest fire. The intensity and location of each inflammatory outbreak varies. It doesn't produce "hard symptoms" that can be objectively observed, like a fractured bone or gallstone. It reveals itself through an ever-changing array of painful, often debilitating "soft symptoms" such as fatigue, brain fog, general body pain, and depression. As you'll see in the stories of my patients, there's nothing "soft" about the experience of these symptoms at all. They can worsen to a catastrophic degree, putting college students in wheelchairs and ruining the careers of fast-track professionals who had rarely been sick before.

Going to a doctor who misses the diagnosis can mean years of needless suffering. Although rheumatoid arthritis, the first autoimmune disease acknowledged by medical science, was recognized in 1950, and others have been discovered since, my clinical practice has convinced me that new autoimmune diseases triggered by infections that specifically target the nervous system have become epidemic in recent years.

Doctors with other specialties tend to be completely unaware of this possibility. Those who don't dismiss their patients' complaints entirely make the mistake of suppressing one symptom after another with drugs, only to see the underlying inflammation flare out of control elsewhere. They're completely mystified about what's going on. So many of my patients have endured frustrated doctors who blatantly doubt their symptoms and even accuse them of exaggerating.

At best, they have found a doctor who arbitrarily decided that one symptom was the problem. One symptom is never the problem with autoimmune disease. The underlying inflammation is the problem, and it can go anywhere in the body it pleases, laying one symptom on top of the next. Each layer must be resolved in turn until the inflammation stops cropping up somewhere else. But if you stop when the symptoms subside, it's like walking away from a forest fire when the trees have stopped burning, but there are still smoldering embers in the grove. The fire isn't out. It will flare up again.

In a situation like this, it's easy to understand why so many people show up at my office feeling discouraged and wondering if there's any hope. After years of tests and treatments, they have thought that it was over time and again. Their blood tests were normal. Their scans were fine. Everything seemed to be normal. Then the slightest change brought the fires of inflammation roaring back. It didn't take much to set it off. It was only a surprise because nobody was watching the embers.

In my office, we always check for the embers of inflammation lingering in the brain, confusing the immune system until it starts attacking its own body. We specialize in interpreting symptoms in the context of the whole person and getting to the cause of the problem. It's essential to not only eliminate each of the pre-existing conditions that have made your body more vulnerable to getting an autoimmune disease from an infection, but also to actively treat the immune system itself so it can function normally again.

Our patients often come to us exasperated that so few of the experts they have sought out – for many years and often at great expense – are able to understand the true nature of their condition and return them to good health.

To make matters worse, most doctors don't realize that there is an entirely new set of autoimmune diseases emerging that are triggered by infections. As a result, they treat only a few of the symptoms and never trace it back to the source: the infection. They also don't realize the importance of addressing the factors that weakened the immune system in the first place and are setting the body up to go haywire and start attacking itself: sleep deficit, gut imbalance, toxic overload, and lingering emotional traumas.

Many patients have been told they have chronic fatigue syndrome or fibromyalgia, as if that explained everything. But it doesn't. Because they also have trouble with their memory and ability to concentrate. How does chronic fatigue explain the fact that they used to be doing demanding jobs or excelling in graduate school and now they have to read a paragraph ten times to understand it? How does it explain the fact that they used to be in vigorous good health and suddenly everything changed?

Now they're mired in a low-grade to severely disabling yuck. They feel crappy all the time. By night, they sleep poorly. By day, they take more and more pills for more and more inexplicable aches or pains. Their lab tests come out normal, but things keep getting worse. They're rightfully worried. Yet their doctor can't imagine what the problem is, so she has exactly the wrong response: "But you look great!"

Life has gotten smaller fairly abruptly in just the last few years. They see they're going down the wrong road, but don't know the way back.

In my practice, we know the way. We accompany people on their journey back to good health all the time. Because not everyone can come to my office in McLean, Virginia, and work with my team, I'm writing this book to share as much as

I possibly can about the process so you can help yourself. As a well-informed patient, you will be better able to know exactly what's happening and make the changes you need.

You will still need a doctor to order lab tests and sometimes prescribe certain medications. If you can find a good doctor who understands autoimmune disease and is willing to work with you as an informed patient, you will benefit from having them as a medical advocate.

As much as we might all wish it would, the change won't happen overnight, but you can begin your return to vibrant health right away.

On our website, there is a short quiz called *The Short Form 36 (SF-36)* that serves as an objective check for the state of your physical and mental health. It can help you and your physician understand how sick you are. You're welcome to go there now and get immediate feedback as to whether your symptoms suggest that a more thorough investigation is needed.

https://kaplanclinic.com/sf36/

AUTOIMMUNITY

There are more than 100 autoimmune diseases where the immune system attacks its own body.[2] In America alone, autoimmunity impacts one in 20 adults.[3] With so many distracting symptoms, a diagnosis of "autoimmunity" can easily slip through the cracks.[4]

Yet the testing for some of them is unreliable, making them hard to diagnose with any certainty. Others are so rare that doctors don't think to test for them. Most are spread across a variety of specialties, so it's hard to find one doctor who puts the whole picture together. Even though inflammatory bowel disease, rheumatoid arthritis, Crohn's disease, lupus, Hashimoto's, and Graves' are all major autoimmune diseases, they are usually listed separately as completely different, unrelated conditions.[5]

When the major autoimmune diseases are counted together, there up to 50 million cases of autoimmunity – as many as cancer and heart disease combined.[6]

What's more, there are signs that we are on the brink of a dramatic increase in autoimmunity. According to a study published by the National Institutes of Health (NIH) on April 7, 2020, there has been a 50 percent increase in the most common biomarker of autoimmunity (antinuclear antibodies, ANA) in the last 25 years.[7]

INFECTION TRIGGERS AUTOIMMUNITY

This new set of autoimmune diseases triggered by infections complicates things. Because the research is just emerging, doctors who are accustomed to looking for the conventional markers for autoimmune diseases don't always make the connection to infections.

Environmental triggers, particularly bacteria, viruses, and other infectious pathogens, play a major role in the development of autoimmune diseases. They can initiate or exacerbate autoimmunity.[8]

One study showed that identical twins only developed autoimmunity when they had both a genetic proclivity and an environmental trigger (such as an infection).[9]

Some researchers speculate that the body attacks normal cells because the antibodies produced in response to infections resemble viruses and bacteria. Others think that the infections themselves damage the immune system.[10]

The virus that causes mumps and measles has been linked to Type 1 diabetes.[11] Multiple sclerosis (MS), rheumatoid arthritis (suspected to be caused by herpes and candida),[12] lupus and

Guillain-Barré syndrome can all be provoked by Epstein-Barr. But since the infections often occur long before the symptoms of autoimmunity appear, few doctors make the connection.[13]

Ideally, thoroughly eliminating the infection would put an end to autoimmunity, once it has developed. That would be the most compelling proof. Acute arthritis, for example, is often alleviated by successfully treating Lyme disease.

In my practice, we have seen dramatic improvements in the lives of my patients once the infection is completely gone.

> Marsha, an athlete and mother of three had Lyme and multiple viral infections. She was disabled by irritable bowel syndrome (IBS), heart palpitations, chronic fatigue, joint pain, numbness, and other irritating nerve symptoms that would come and go. Now she is back to running marathons and recently became a mother of four.
>
> Ellen came to see me in her 20s. Shortly after graduating from college, she began suffering from headaches and joint pain. Within two years, she developed severe stomach pains and diarrhea. Her weight dropped from a healthy 128 pounds to a life-threatening 85 pounds. Ellen had Crohn's disease. The probable cause was an infection called mycobacterium avium.[14] After treating the root infection, then each of the issues that had set her up for autoimmune disease, we took active steps to calm her immune system. Today, Ellen's symptoms are completely gone. She has fallen in love, married, and has a gorgeous baby boy.
>
> Chris, a general contractor, developed a severe gastrointestinal infection while traveling overseas. When he began to experience increasing muscle weakness in his legs, he was diagnosed with Guillain-Barré syn-

drome, an autoimmune disease that causes paralysis. It begins in the legs but can ultimately paralyze the entire body. The bacteria that had caused both his gastrointestinal infection and triggered the autoimmune disease, Guillain-Barré, was campylobacter jejuni.[15] Once the infection was treated, Chris steadily recovered his strength. He now owns his own company and manages major construction projects.

Unfortunately, it is often more complicated. Pathogens can continue to cause a disease even after the original infection has been completely eliminated.[16] And sometimes a single infection can trigger several different autommunity (autoimmune) diseases.[17]

IMPACT

The average person with autoimmunity sees five doctors over three-and-a-half years before they receive an accurate diagnosis.[18]

Along the way they may have been diagnosed with conditions like chronic fatigue syndrome (ME/CFS), fibromyalgia, post-treatment Lyme syndrome, chronic depression, IBS, or even obsessive-compulsive disorder. The problem with these very real diagnoses is that they are the end of the exploration of why you are sick when they should be only the beginning.

Many of my patients have described the relief they experienced when someone finally identified the problem. A diagnostic label from a medical professional can feel like validation after months or years of uncertainty. It can feel great to know you're not imagining things and being a hypochondriac. But it's far more important to find a doctor who sees the big picture, understands the implications of your condition, and knows how to resolve it.

People suffering from autoimmunity often experience extreme states of debilitation. It's not uncommon to be unable to work or go to school. This can derail financial security and interrupt the natural course of their lives.

Yet most of the time, they don't particularly look sick. Their own loved ones lose patience and wonder if they're exaggerating or just not trying hard enough. When a disease is virtually invisible, it is even harder to identify.[19]

The increasing tendency for doctors to specialize increases the challenge of finding a physician who can recognize what's going on with a disease that encompasses many specialties like autoimmunity.

Each one simply addresses their own specialty and, at best, refers patients to specialists for any other symptoms. But if that happens, who will see – and treat – the whole?

A psychiatrist may prescribe medications for the symptoms of depression, anxiety disorder, behavioral disorder, or obsessive disorder. But it is the truly rare psychiatrist who would connect a case of Epstein-Barr you had last year as the source of your depression, nor are they even aware, in most cases, that an infection could lie at the root of your symptoms.

As autoimmunity ramps up, the symptoms start piling on top of one another like lemmings tumbling over a cliff into the sea. An assortment unique to each individual emerges, including fatigue, poor digestion, headaches, sleep, brain fog, pain, heart palpitations, inability to stand, blackouts, and any other symptoms that can be caused by the inflammation of the brain that is creating them.

The inflammation itself is frequently set off by an infection, then compounded by trauma and toxins.

Depression, anxiety, chronic fatigue, chronic pain, and many other issues are the consequence of inflammation in the brain. The inflammation in the brain is the immune system's response to tissue damage from infections, toxins, and other assaults. These assaults include chronic stress and other emotional traumas.

It is essential then to treat not just the illness – with its infections, physical traumas, and toxins – but the whole body and the immune system itself.

The acquired immune system is our specialized defense force. It is the force that builds antibodies to not only fight specific illnesses, but it also remembers the attackers and keeps us safe from being invaded again by the same armies of germs. It is also the force that, when sick and traumatized, can get very confused and begin to attack us. It's a condition called autoimmunity, self against self.

Although it is acknowledged that there is an "autoimmune epidemic," most doctors focus on conventional autoimmune diseases, such as rheumatoid arthritis, lupus, inflammatory bowel disease, multiple sclerosis, Type 1 diabetes mellitus, Guillain-Barré syndrome, psoriasis, and others, while the number of people suffering from new autoimmune diseases is growing by the day.

Approximately ten percent of Americans may be suffering with undiagnosed autoimmunity. The revolution coming in medicine is that damage to our acquired immune system is far more common and, indeed, is the underlying problem in a huge number of conditions as varied as Pediatric Acute-onset Neuropsychiatric disorder (PANS), Pediatric Autoimmune Neuropsychiatric Disorder Associated with Streptococcus (PANDAS), depression, fibromyalgia, chronic fatigue syndrome, Postural Orthostatic Tachycardia Syndrome (POTS), multiple sclerosis, and many more. Autoimmunity caused from physical or emotional trauma, toxins, infections, or a combination of these assaults may be the most important insight into chronic disease of the 21st century.

Damage to our cell powerhouses – the mitochondria – are also a part of this problem-causing chronic illness and impairment of our immune systems. This concept of mitochondrial damage, championed by Dr. Robert Naviaux, which he calls the "cell danger response," is rapidly being recognized as another crucial element to total recovery.[20]

To heal, you must identify and treat all of the issues that have caused your immune system to become sick, but failure to also treat your immune system keeps you from fully recovering. Worse yet, this leaves you primed for the next assault that can send you cascading down into permanent disability.

THE SET-UP

Your immune system is devoted to protecting you from infections. The only reason it will not do that is if something else is impairing its ability to function.

The top four reasons for this impairment are: unhealthy sleep, abused gut, environmental toxins, and emotional trauma. When your immune system has been undermined by these conditions, your body is set up for trouble. Once you get an infection, your odds of developing autoimmune disease have greatly increased

SET-UP + INFECTION = AUTOIMMUNE DISEASE

SOLUTION

All of these issues are neuroinflammatory. What started out as an infection can quickly become a serious immune challenge. To recover, you will need to find the infections, then find and treat each of the other issues that set you up: first the toxins, then the gut, then the trauma, then the sleep. As we tick these things off one at a time, we then treat the immune system itself to calm it down and return it to its optimal state. Only then will you be free from autoimmune disease.

1. Find the infections
2. Eliminate the infections
3. Treat the toxins, gut, trauma, and sleep issues
4. Calm the immune system

In this book, I will give you a comprehensive method for healing, a new way of thinking about and approaching the problem, and tools that will allow you to figure out whether you have these issues and, if you do, will show you how to fix them.

You're going to have to take charge because most physicians don't think like this. We're too siloed into specialties in the medical field today. If you go to the orthopedist who specializes in shoulder pain, but your pain is in the fifth digit of your right hand, you're in the wrong doctor's office. You'll have to go to a fifth-digit specialist. In the chapters that follow, you will be given the tools you need to become your own best advocate for your health.

CHAPTER 2

—

HOW YOUR IMMUNE SYSTEM CAN TURN ON YOU

Our bodies come equipped with an incredible defense system so finely tuned that it is instantly aware of the least incursion – down to the microscopic level. Threats are immediately identified and attacked, then put on a kind of immunological "watch list" in case they ever dare to come back again. Our immune system erects phenomenal barriers to protect us from the millions of potential pathogens we touch, ingest, or inhale every single day.

Our immune system is like a supercomputer going full bore 24/7. This is the same system that can give you back perfectly smooth skin after you've ripped it off to the bone or restore vigorous health to your lungs after you've come down with a bad case of pneumonia. It's always got your back and can't bear to let you down, even if it dies trying.

Made up of an incredibly complex array of cells that protect us from invasion and assault, the immune system is perhaps the most complex system in our bodies, apart from our brains. In some ways, it's almost too quick, too responsive, and too powerful. We now know that our remarkable immune system – the most perfect system ever devised – can kill us.

Across America there is a growing epidemic of mysterious illnesses. Sometimes they go by names like chronic fatigue syndrome, fibromyalgia, chronic Lyme, chronic pain syndrome, depression, PANS, mast cell activation syndrome, or chronic daily headaches. More often, one part of the illness is treated – more or less effectively, often temporarily – and doctors dismiss the other symptoms as if they were unrelated. This temptation is easy to understand, since the patients come in with multiple complaints.

Doctors typically do what they're most familiar with, handing out prescriptions that block the symptoms. This masks the problem and often makes it worse. At best, it completely ignores the underlying disease.

At The Kaplan Center, I've spent 30 years treating people struggling with these symptoms. What I've learned is that if you block the symptoms without treating the underlying issues, another symptom will appear. That's how we know the inflammation has reached the brain.

Brain inflammation is not an event, but a process. It is the result of multiple points of origin. Each one has fed into the other, increasing the inflammation. Whether it shows up as headaches, allergies, or heart palpitations depends on the individual.

If you take non-steroidal anti-inflammatory drugs (NSAIDs) to block your headache pain, the inflammation will simply crop up somewhere else. Since NSAIDs also disrupt the balance of bacteria in your gut, maybe the inflammation will manifest in gas or an irritable bowel. Maybe your allergies will get worse. You may think there's just more pollen in the air, but if you weren't in a state of inflammation – taking pills that make things worse – the higher pollen may not have affected you at all.

The trouble is most doctors aren't thinking like medical detectives. They don't know to look at the whole body for signs of inflammation, although one symptom after another is showing up.

They don't realize that unless they treat the disease, not the symptoms, your body can develop a state of constant inflammation that can destroy your resilience, make your life miserable on a daily basis, and ultimately set you up for nearly every degenerative disease on record – osteoarthritis, amyotrophic lateral sclerosis (ALS), dementia, MS, Parkinson's, Alzheimer's – to name a few.

In this book, you will learn how your immune system is working for you around the clock and what's going on in your body behind the scenes when these symptoms start cropping up and the doctors can't find anything wrong.

UNEARTHING ROOT CAUSES

Our realization that the innate immune system is responsible for many chronic conditions that have long eluded medical science was a game changer that allowed us to finally focus on root causes, rather than attempting to treat symptoms with dismal results. Suddenly, we had new places to look when patients showed up with unexplained symptoms. Anything that potentially caused brain inflammation was suspect:

- **Toxins** (heavy metals, molds, pesticides)
- **Traumas** (physical, psychological)
- **Infections** (tick-borne diseases, mononucleosis, bacteria, viruses)
- **Gut imbalances** (yeast, bacterial overgrowth, leaky gut)
- **Loss of oxygen to the brain** (sleep apnea)
- **Loss of blood to the brain** (POTS)

The results were remarkable. Patients who had suffered for years with disabling pain, fatigue, and episodes that appeared to be seizures were symptom-free once we eliminated mold toxicity and Lyme infections from their bodies. In my own practice, I have been delighted to see that the treatment of chronic mono eliminates chronic fatigue syndrome, and the treatment of sleep apnea eliminates chronic daily headaches.

THE IMPOSSIBLE HAPPENS

The brain and nervous system of the human body regulate the functions of our organs, glands, and tissues so that our temperature, blood sugar, fluid levels, blood pressure, and other functions maintain a dependably steady state we call *homeostasis*.

The work our bodies do 24/7 behind the scenes is an unequivocal marvel. Our muscular system alone consists of 650 muscles, allowing us to do many things we take for granted like standing, moving, and generating heat or blood flow. Under our skin are more than 206 long, short, flat, and oddly shaped bones, supported by joints, cartilage, and tendons that support and protect our most essential organs.[21] Beneath our skulls are 86 billion neurons connected by trillions of synapses[22] and blood vessels that would stretch for 100,000 miles.[23] Every single day, we take over 20,000 breaths.[24] Even though we'd never be able to keep count, our hearts beat more than 42 million times every year.[25]

As magnificent as the human body is, it also wields an almost inconceivable power to shift that vital homeostasis in an instant. Normally, that power is used to protect and defend us. But when mistakes are made, the consequences can be devastating.

One of these mistakes is a leading cause of death and disability in America. A simple error in identification causes the immune system to mistake its body's tissues for the foreign invaders and attack. Suddenly, we become our own worst enemy.

The carnage that results in the body from these attacks of the immune system is known as *autoimmunity*. There are now more than 100 known variations of this disease, depending on which systems in the body are most affected. The alarming cascade of destruction that occurs when the body turns on itself has become so prevalent that it now affects almost 24 million Americans.[26]

In the late 1800s, these attacks were dismissed as impossible by the renowned medical pioneer, Dr. Paul Ehrlich, who was convinced that the body had a powerful safeguard in place to prevent such attacks: an innate aversion to immunological self-destruction. He called it *horror autotoxicus* ("horror of self-toxification").[27]

Ehrlich himself would have been horrified to learn that his reputation had given so much weight to his words that it blocked medical progress on this strange, counter-intuitive disease for nearly 50 years.

Even before winning the Nobel Prize in 1908 and being nominated again in 1913, Ehrlich was a shining star in medical science.[28] He made countless contributions in fields as diverse as immunology, histology, hematology, microbiology, pharmacology, and oncology, even developing early chemotherapy.[29] He simply couldn't imagine why the body would turn on itself. As a result, immunological research in medicine was replaced by a chemical orientation that prevented an entire generation of doctors from understanding what was really going on.[30]

It's a good reminder that what seems to be true is often colored by our preconceptions. Even the giants of medicine can make mistakes that do harm to medicine, just as our immune systems can make mistakes that harm our own bodies. When we forget the fundamental uncertainty of our world or try to hide from it with false certainties, we make an even graver mistake. It's far better to recognize that not knowing everything gives us endless possibilities for hope.

THE TRAUMATIZED IMMUNE SYSTEM

From the moment we emerged from our mothers' wombs, our lives have relied on our strong, capable immune system. It protects us from infections, helps us heal from trauma, prevents us from getting cancer.

Without it, we die. But if it goes into overdrive, it can kill us.

Our immune system is vastly complex with multiple back-up and fail-safe mechanisms. At its most basic, it is two systems: the innate immune system (the first responders) and the acquired immune system (the specialists).

The innate immune system sends out the first responders. It acts as our first line of defense and kills off any invading pathogens (viruses, bacteria, parasites). At the same time, it acts as a demolition crew cleaning up the mess from whatever damage was done. Next, it calls in the repair crews to repair the damage. When the crisis is over, the innate immune system stands down and waits, alert and ready to respond to the next threat to your health.

The acquired (also known as adaptive) immune system is our second line of defense. It specializes in attacking specific bugs with antibodies. When we are immunized against diseases, it is a way to introduce our immune systems to a new enemy. It gives these internal warriors time to develop the training, strategies, and experience for defeating this enemy should it ever come back in larger numbers. Armed and ready, your adaptive immune system will be better able to kill off chickenpox, polio, tetanus, or meningitis in the future – before we even feel a thing.

When our systems are overloaded, the strain can be too much for either one of our immune systems. The first responders are also likely to be the first to become exhausted, then traumatized, then hyper-reactive.

We now know that the innate immune system can develop a type of PTSD. Even after these first responders have eliminated the mold toxins, infections, or other foreign invaders, they can't relax. If they were people, we'd say that they seemed jumpy, paranoid and hyper-vigilant, and needed to cut back on the caffeine for a few days. When it happens in the immune system, we need to intervene, helping to reduce inflammation in the brain, so they can return to their normal, resting state – always vigilant, but less prone to attack for no reason.

Total recovery requires not only treating the original cause of the fire but treating the first responders as well.

Imagine a group of fire fighters who have fought a massive fire that took immense effort to control. Every time they thought they had the fire contained, it flared up behind another wall or ceiling. They fought this fire for days and are now not just exhausted, but traumatized by the experience, hyper alert for any new flare-ups. You can imagine that in their concern to make sure the building was safe they might get a little too aggressive knocking down walls, looking any and everywhere for remnants of the fire. This is what happens to the first responders in our brains.

THE WRONG QUESTIONS

For too long, we have been asking the wrong questions about most chronic illnesses and as a result, we have been focused on the symptoms and not the cause. The consequences of this have been staggering in terms of suffering and economic costs.

Western medicine is great at illnesses with clear causes and effects. You get a strep throat, we give you an antibiotic, and you are cured.

With high blood pressure, on the other hand, we do not actually know the cause. But we can measure it objectively. More importantly, we have a whole pharmacy of medications to control the symptom, though not to cure the problem.

Pain, depression, fatigue, anxiety, brain fog, as well as noise and sound sensitivity, are things you feel but we cannot measure. We will run tests. But if the tests come back normal, your physician, just like you, will start to feel helpless. The response is usually empathy, but sometimes denial by the physician that there is anything wrong with you.

When I was on the advisory committee for chronic fatigue syndrome (ME/CFS) at the Department of Health and Human Services, I heard hundreds of people testify how they had been dismissed by physicians. Many were told they were crazy, just faking, and were left unable to work and unable to get disability because their physicians refused to acknowledge their illness.

Unfortunately, in this situation, your symptoms are virtually invisible to medical science. We can measure the damage from a heart attack. We cannot measure your experience of crippling pain or fatigue.

THE MODERN TRAGEDY

When it comes to treatment, the results have been disastrous. Our blind attempts to treat pain that we don't understand created the opioid epidemic that killed more than 70,000 Americans in 2017 alone.[31]

Unfortunately, all too often, when your physician cannot identify the cause of your symptoms, they may decide the symptoms themselves are the problem and recommend surgery, destroy a nerve, or perform a procedure in the hopes of helping you, but end up making things worse.

People suffering with chronic fatigue, fibromyalgia, headaches, pain, and a number of other chronic conditions frequently end up being referred to a psychologist instead of receiving the medical treatment they need. The delay in treatment results in a worsening or spread of the condition, compounded by the stigma of being told the condition is "imaginary." This egregious waste of time and resources would be far better spent searching for an answer to the physical problem.

At the same time, there may well be a psychological component amplifying the problem. Stress and trauma, such as early childhood abuse, can certainly provoke brain inflammation. These early childhood traumas may start a smoldering fire that, when you encounter additional assailants such as toxins or an infection, flare into a blazing inferno that leads to chronic pain, chronic depression, incapacitating fatigue, and disability. While addressing these early traumas is important, it is more important to understand that these assaults are actually doing physical damage to the brain.

WHAT IS THE IMMUNE SYSTEM?

In the brain, the most important cell of the innate immune system is the microglia, which I wrote about extensively in *Total Recovery*. Since that book came out, there has been extensive research on a second innate immune cell in the brain called mast cells.

Mast cells are found in the brain and all over the body. When stimulated, they release numerous chemical messengers. The most famous of these is histamine. Histamine is what causes hives and allergic reactions. It can set off an allergic asthma attack.

You may not know it, but whenever you take an antihistamine, you are actually trying to quiet down the reaction of your mast cells.

Anaphylactic reactions are also caused by mast cells. If you are allergic to shellfish and accidentally eat a shrimp, your skin may break out with a rash, your blood pressure may drop, and your airways may swell, making it hard for you to breathe. An anaphylactic reaction can kill you. And it is brought to you compliments of your own hyper-reactive mast cells.

It seems that mast cells, like microglia, can develop a type of PTSD. When they become over-reactive, they can do a lot of damage. The new condition that results is called mast cell activation syndrome (MCAS) and it can wreak havoc with your health.

Symptoms of MCAS may appear as chronic fatigue, fibromyalgia, chronic pelvic pain, depression, vomiting, or diarrhea. It has even shown up as the underlying cause of psychological disorders that expressed themselves in cutting behavior.[32]

Like microglia, mast cells are a blunt instrument in protecting us from outside attacks. They communicate with the acquired immune system, which is a lot more nuanced and specific. The acquired immune system is the part of the immune system that makes antibodies. Antibodies are like soldiers who are trained to fight and protect us from very specific threats.

Let's imagine that your house was invaded by ravaging raccoons. The pest control agency you hired to protect your house against termites and other bugs is not trained in handling raccoons specifically. These are clever raccoons, and you need a specialist. So, you go out and hire the guys who specialize in eliminating ravaging raccoons. These guys are raccoon warriors, and they will eliminate and continue to protect your house from ravaging raccoons.

With these warriors on the job, there is no way any pesky raccoon is ever getting back into your house. These guys are spectacular at eliminating raccoons, but so highly trained that they aren't very effective against anything else. So, if your house is invaded by cats, the raccoon warriors are not even going to lift an eyebrow while the cats invade and take over your house, peeing on your house plants, eating your lasagna, leaving hair balls everywhere, etc. Okay, I have wandered into a personal issue here, but you get the idea.

The other thing you need to know about the anti-raccoon warriors is that sometimes they are so highly specialized that while they will protect your house from raccoons with brown eyes, if the raccoons have blue eyes, they may not bother with them any more than the cats.

When you get a flu shot, you cause your body to produce very specific warriors (antibodies) that protect you from getting the flu virus. "Flu" is actually not a single virus, but a family of viruses. The flu vaccine we give you is designed to only create warriors who will guard against certain members of the flu family. Thus, like the raccoons, if you are attacked by the blue-eyed flu family and we immunized you against the brown-eyed flu family, you will get the flu. So, in sum, the antibodies we make are designed to kill very specific bugs. Sometimes the protection can last a lifetime, such as with measles and mumps, while with other bugs like the flu, the protection is for a much shorter time.

IT'S THE IMMUNE SYSTEM, STUPID

In my first book *Total Recovery*, I discussed what was, at the time, emerging research that depression was actually a symptom of an inflamed brain. There are, as we have learned, two basic divisions of the immune system – the innate or first responders and the adaptive or specialized immune system. *Total Recovery* looked at the research about the innate immune system's involvement in brain inflammation resulting in the symptoms of depression as well as chronic fatigue and chronic pain.

This idea that depression and other psychiatric disorders, as well as neurological diseases such as Parkinson's disease, multiple sclerosis, and even Alzheimer's disease and conditions such as chronic fatigue syndrome and fibromyalgia, are symptoms of an inflammatory response is extremely important and a major breakthrough in our thinking about these diseases. Each of these conditions certainly has a distinct presentation, most likely secondary to your genetic predisposition, but they also have much more in common than we previously thought.

We now know that our first responder, the innate immune system, is capable of learning. Frankly, we thought for the longest time that the first responders were a bit stupid. Bad things happened to the body, causing the first responders to move in and destroy the invaders, clean up the mess, and call the repair crews. Then they grab a beer, kick back, and watch for the next threat. They responded a little bit differently to bugs than to cell damage from other things, but frankly, were not especially creative in how they handled each situation. The bright guys were the adaptive immune system; they could create specific weapons to destroy specific threats.

Well, the first responders, it turns out, are not quite so stupid after all. They chat on a regular basis with the adaptive immune system and even help keep it regulated.

We now understand that our first responders are capable of learning lessons they pick up from hanging out with the adaptive immune system. What they learn, though, is a bit of a mixed bag and does not always produce the best results.

WHAT THE INNATE IMMUNE SYSTEMS LEARNS

For years, there were reports about how when we gave a vaccine for a specific bug, say small pox, we also noted that people who got the vaccine also saw improvement in allergic reactions and other disease such as measles and even syphilis.[33] These nonspecific effects from a vaccine that should only have offered protection, via our adaptive immune system, to the specific bug it was designed for, turns out to be caused by the effects the vaccine had on our first responders, the innate immune system who wasn't supposed to be teachable.

It now seems that our first responders can "learn" and not only respond to the first bug that attacks us but become hyper-alert to other bugs not related to the first. It's good to know that they're now ready to vigorously protect us from more than one bug. But this hyper-vigilance can result in a low-grade chronic inflammation in our system that wreaks all kinds of havoc, including setting us up for mental illness, chronic pain, chronic fatigue, and neurodegenerative diseases such as Alzheimer's.

This is a different response by the innate immune system than the type of PTSD I have discussed previously, where the innate immune system has been "traumatized" from fighting an extreme or long-standing battle, but the result is to some extent the same.

You end up with an overactive group of first responders that are now part of the problem.

Why is this important? If you know the immune system, and specifically which part of the immune system is facilitating the problem, you can target your treatment to get a much better result.

Also, if you know the immune system is mediating the problem, you now start trying to understand what activated the immune system in the first place and can target your treatment to fix that problem first. Toxins vs. Bugs, for instance.

What about the acquired immune system?

First, let's stand back and ask: "What causes the acquired immune system to make mistakes that are truly life-altering and life-threatening?"

Certainly genetics, but genetics are less destiny than an indication of what is possible. After all, about 30 percent of people have the genes that could cause them to develop celiac disease, but only 3 percent ever develop the disease.[34] So, genes unquestionably play a role, but, as we shall see, so do other things like bacterial and viral infections, your childhood, your stress level, the health of your intestinal tract, your sleep patterns, and your exposure to toxins such as mold or heavy metals. There are undoubtedly many other triggers too, but we already have strong evidence for these.

It is well-established now that many of these triggers can ignite the autoimmunity of the conventional autoimmune disorders. Crohn's disease has been linked to an infection called mycobacterium avium.[35] Infections with EBV (the virus that causes mono) may be linked to the development of multiple sclerosis.[36] A high-stress childhood increases the risk of developing autoimmunity,[37] and the heath of your gut is intimately related to the health of your immune system in conditions such as Type 1 diabetes and rheumatoid arthritis.[38]

EXCITING BREAKTHROUGHS

It's not just our thinking about the innate immune system that has changed radically in the last few years. The smart guys in the acquired immune system apparently have a few more lessons to teach us. It seems that the acquired immune system also makes mistakes.

We have known for decades now that our immune system can attack us. Over 23 million people suffer with diseases such as rheumatoid arthritis, systemic lupus erythematosus (SLE), multiple sclerosis, and Crohn's disease – all the result of our acquired immune system gone rogue. And these are only the "conventional autoimmunities." We're about to go way beyond that.[39]

As our understanding of the acquired immune system has grown, so has our arsenal of therapies to treat the consequences of these devastating diseases. With powerful disease-modifying antirheumatic drugs (DMARDs), we are now able to control the symptoms of many autoimmune diseases. Unfortunately, our approach to managing these diseases is still fairly primitive. As the name implies, DMARDs modify, but do not cure the diseases. And one of their unfortunate side effects is an increased risk of life-threating infections and certain cancers. Nonetheless, these drugs have been a godsend for many patients.

Another massive breakthrough is our new ability to weaponize the immune system to fight cancer. Immunotherapies are now being used with spectacular results. They treat a multitude of cancers, from cancers of the blood to cancers of the brain. This is truly one of the most exciting fields in medicine and holds promise for not only new treatments, but possibly a cure for many cancers. It's all very exciting for people with conventional autoimmune diseases. But what if you have a new autoimmunity?

NEW AUTOIMMUNITY

No trauma plunged Jenn into chronic daily headaches. No specific illness set them off. She had never had chronic headaches before. One day when she was still in high school, Jenn just woke up with a headache and it never went away.

The usual over-the-counter medications did nothing to stop them. When her local physician didn't help, she began what turned into years of extensive workups and treatments by the best doctors at one of the best headache centers in the country. But she still had headaches.

Remarkably, she managed to complete her education at a top university and landed a significant job at a prominent consulting firm in Washington, D.C. Smart and very personable, a natural networker with a knack for clarifying company goals, identifying impediments to progress, and getting people to work together, Jenn proved to be a rapidly rising star.

Few people knew that she was achieving so much while suffering from nonstop headaches for 15 years. As time passed, the accumulating years and her increasing age started tipping the scales against her.

The pain was getting significantly worse all the time. It wasn't just headaches anymore. The head pain had begun to spread throughout her body. The stress of maintaining a high-functioning career under the weight of constant pain was starting to wear her down. Some days she experienced such crushing fatigue and outright exhaustion that she would fall asleep for 18 hours.

Her body seemed to be moving into a state of near-constant hypersensitivity. Light and sound that had always been perfectly acceptable became hard to endure. The positive, can-do attitude that had always supported her through life was sliding into an emotional pit of depression and anxiety, despite her best efforts to fend it off. To make matters worse, she couldn't think straight half the time! Brain fog was taking more and more days away from her.

It took a while for her to accept what was happening. She kept trying to push through it at work, but the days she had to miss were starting to add up. The very idea of taking a medical leave of absence terrified her. It felt like resignation. It was as if it meant that she was succumbing to this mysterious illness, admitting defeat. But eventually, she had no choice.

Determined to find answers, Jenn turned all her attention to finding new doctors, new medical centers, and new treatments, but her health continued to decline.

When I met Brenda, she was in her late 40s, well-dressed, smart, and charming. She, too, had a very successful career as vice president in a financial firm. Traveling constantly and working 60-hour weeks was the norm for her job.

Her prospects for continued success and prosperity had been on the rise, until a trip abroad changed everything. A deeply religious woman, she had gone on a pilgrimage to Europe with her husband and their priest. She had been healthy on the trip, but within two weeks of returning home she developed severe fatigue and a headache. Nothing had been the same since.

Even as I was taking her history, it was apparent to me that she was much sicker than first impressions would suggest. Her confident, professional presentation belied the fact that she was suffering from severe fatigue, daily headaches, and overall pain. Not only was she unable to focus on anything – a skill she had always relied on – but any attempt to concentrate made her headache and fatigue dramatically worse!

"I've seen pretty much all the -ologists," Brenda told me. Pages of medical records listed neurologists, immunologists, gastroenterologists, and other specialists of various flavors – over 20 physicians in all. Their initial diagnosis had been mononucleosis, but that had proved to be unhelpful. Despite being hospitalized at a major medical center at one point, then spending three weeks in a multidisciplinary program to treat her headaches, she was no better off than before.

Eager to return to work, she negotiated a change to a less demanding position that required less travel and fewer hours, but to her dismay, even that proved to be too much. Less than two years from the onset of her illness, Brenda had to go on disability, leaving the position she loved and had worked so hard to achieve.

Like Jenn, Brenda developed a sensitivity to noise and sound that required her to frequently retreat to the cool, dark, quiet of her bedroom. She became despondent and depressed to the point of requiring hospitalization for the depression. Things were getting worse. Despite all of the medical attention she'd received, she did not even have a diagnosis when I saw her.

For Julian, the world came crashing in even sooner – when he was a sophomore in high school. Charismatic with a winning smile and a great sense of humor, Julian had always been a natural athlete and honors student, well-liked by all his peers. Then as his father tells it, "A switch went off and it sent him into a downward spiral."

Julian developed bizarre and terrifying mood swings: violent outbursts, screaming fits, and crying without provocation. His parents were stunned. Not only was this behavior completely unlike anything they'd ever seen in their son before, but it was also completely irrational and extreme.

One minute he would suffer a complete breakdown, curled up under his bed sobbing and tearing at his chest, the next he would be yelling, throwing furniture, and breaking things in a rage. The storm could last for an hour or more before it subsided. Exhausted, Julian would calm down and fall asleep for several hours, then wake up smiling and friendly like his usual self, only to meltdown and start all over again.

Alarmed, his parents rushed him to the emergency room at a children's hospital the first time it happened. Doctors there hospitalized him immediately in the psych ward.

Told that his issues were psychological, Julian was given medications for mood and anxiety disorders before he was released. But the episodes continued despite the medications. To make matters worse, Julian developed an eating disorder in response to a severely distorted image of his body, called body dysmorphia. When his weight dropped to 108 pounds from 140, his parents enrolled him in an inpatient eating disorder program. Six months later, there were signs that the medications were having some effect on Julian's moods, but he was still not healthy enough to return to school.

What was missed in all three of these patients was that their plunge into new autoimmunity had started with infections. Each one of them had contracted Lyme disease and other tick-borne infections that lit the fuse on the debilitating explosion of symptoms that followed.

Distracted by the complexity of their cases, doctors failed to identify the origin of their illness. In each case, there were plenty of distractions to go around. Apart from constant pain, Jenn had both mold toxicity and hypermobility syndrome. Along with her severe fatigue and headaches, Brenda suffered from PTSD, depression, a severe imbalance of intestinal flora, sleep apnea, and a genetic defect that not only impaired her ability to assimilate B vitamins but also made her body resistant to our treatments for depression. On top of his emotional pyrotechnics, Julian also had chronic mono and chronic strep.

Thanks to a tick bite, their immune systems had become a major part of the problem and brought on new autoimmunity.

The old-school approach of one infection, one antibiotic fails people with this condition.

In all chronic diseases, inflammation is the underlying problem. That inflammation may have a multitude of causes – including tick bites. To achieve a cure, we need to identify and treat them all.

Unlike conventional autoimmune disorders, there is not yet conventional agreement on the testing and treatment of new autoimmune disorders. Nevertheless, there is a clear process for identifying underlying problems and treatments that work. In the chapters that follow, I will walk you through the steps.

As we've said in Chapter 1, conventional autoimmune disorders are notoriously hard to treat. The good news is that with new autoimmune disorders, there is a high probability of cure.

—

CHAPTER 3

HOW INFECTIONS TRIP OFF AUTOIMMUNITY

- *When our bodies produce antibodies that attack our own cells, it is called autoimmunity.*
- *Four ways infections cause our immune systems to turn on us.*
- *The five most common infections that trigger autoimmunity.*

For too many people, hidden infections are where it all begins. Once their symptoms are labeled as fibromyalgia, chronic fatigue syndrome, POTS, depression, or anxiety, physicians all too often stop looking for the cause. While this provides labels that are acceptable to insurance companies, it also results in misguided treatments, leaving tens of millions of people sick and disabled.

Hidden infections can have devastating consequences. In *The Lady's Handbook for Her Mysterious Illness*, Sarah Ramey describes a common experience shared by patients (like the one she calls "Jane") when they attempt to describe their symptoms with a conventional doctor.

> The interaction begins very seriously, a furious scribbling of notes, a furrowing of the brow, a lot

of nodding. The usual diseases are ruled out and Jane confirms she has been tested, twice, for everything under the sun. Her primary symptoms are severe constipation, distention, and pain in the lower left quadrant of her abdomen. As the doctor pages through her thick medical file, Jane takes the opportunity to share some of the stranger non-bowel symptoms she has experienced – aching in the bones, fatigue, itching, unexplained gynecologic symptoms, memory problems, lower back pain – but the words are scarcely out of her mouth before she wishes she had kept her addenda to herself. She can see the red flags rising behind his eyes, and the note taking slowly tapers off. Before she knows it, where once Sherlock Holmes scribbled furiously, hot on the trail, bent on solving her mystery – he now leans back in his swivel chair, tip of his pen in the corner of his mouth, checking his watch. His look is saturated with understanding, for he has solved the case.

What we have here is not a rare, tropical disease, Watson. What we have here is an unhappy woman, badly in need of an antidepressant.[40]

Now patients not only have a complex disease with a hidden infection that is challenging to identify and defeat, but they are also saddled with the disdain and dismissal of the medical practitioner they were relying on to help. Not only is it counterproductive, but it's also the last thing they need!

Sarah chronicles her own descent into the hellhole of ME/CFS, chronic pelvic pain, fibromyalgia, POTS, and complex regional pain syndrome (CRPS) that devastated her health as a result of a missed infection with courage, brutal honesty, and wry, dark humor. But her life-altering struggle and those of thousands of others could have been avoided if these hidden infections had not been missed.

As I write this book, we are in the midst of a pandemic that was initially missed. Its variants are continuing to evolve. As of January 2022, SARS-CoV-2, the virus that causes Covid-19, has infected more than 75 million Americans and has killed over 888,000 people in the United States alone.

While we have been focused on the horrendous death toll, it is becoming apparent that Covid-19 can also cause a long-term illness that looks a lot like ME/CFS.

Unfortunately, it is still early on in this pandemic. Our resources are rightfully devoted to controlling this disease, caring for the acutely ill, finding better treatments, and continuing to develop vaccines. The early data suggest that we are also going to have to understand how to treat those with long-lasting disease, and the model we are discussing here is going to be crucial in helping people recover.

One of the crucial questions is why some people who contract Covid-19 develop no symptoms at all or recover quickly, while others become severely ill and die. It's already clear that the virus causes the immune system to malfunction, firing its considerable arsenal against healthy tissue instead of the virus itself. Studies already suggest that to resolve the most severe cases of Covid-19 with long-term repercussions, patients might require an immunological reset.[41]

Normally, the immune system reacts to an invasion by producing *cytokines* that provoke inflammation. After their initial assault, the cytokines retreat so the antibodies and T cells can hone in on the virus and destroy it. Viral immunologist Catherine Blish of Stanford University says, "It's normal to develop inflammation during a viral infection. The problem comes when you can't resolve it."[42]

In those who develop severe cases of Covid-19, the normal immune process breaks down, much like it does in autoimmune disease. In this case, the cytokines that responded first never retreat. Antibodies and T cells still rush in to kill the virus, but with so many forces in play, it only raises levels of inflammation, causing what *The New York Times* calls "a wildfire response of inflammation (*that*) may never get snuffed out, even when it's no longer needed." This reaction gives us every reason to believe that Covid-19 has already begun to introduce a whole new version of autoimmune disease.[43]

HOW AUTOIMMUNITY WORKS

As I mentioned earlier, our bodies have both an innate immune system and an acquired immune system. When you hit your head, the innate immune system sends out the first responders to secure the perimeter, stop the damage from spreading, clean up the mess, call in the repair crew, and then stand ready for the next threat. The acquired immune system makes antibodies that fight off and protect you from more complicated threats.

When our bodies produce antibodies that attack our own cells, it is called *autoimmunity*.

Molecular mimicry is a deadly case of mistaken identity. It is one of the leading mechanisms with which an infection or toxin can induce autoimmunity.[44]

If an infection can create enough confusion, our immune system will begin to see our own cells as invaders. The healthy cells in our brain, nervous system, joints, and/or organs suddenly appear to be threats to our health.

Do you remember a time when you went up to someone in the supermarket that you were convinced was your best friend, but when you went to greet her, realized at the last second that it was a complete stranger? There were enough visual clues, her height and build, hair color, and perhaps the way she carried herself, that you could have sworn it was your friend. We have all done this at one time or another and in general, aside from a moment of awkward embarrassment, it's not a big deal.

The same thing can and does happen to our immune system. A bug or some chemical has enough molecular similarity to our own cells that our immune system mistakes the cells in our own body as an invader that needs to be killed and launches an attack on us. This is not an embarrassing moment. This is the beginning of a disaster.

1. Epigenetics

Epigenetics refers to the impact of the environment on our DNA. Infections, toxins, stress, healthy habits, exercise, smoking, alcohol, drugs, pollution, and countless other factors affect the way our genes affect us.

Used in this way, the term epigenetics has only been around since the 1990s, so it is still an emerging science. Since the Greek prefix word *epi* means "on top of," it was added to describe the way our environment creates an extra layer of instructions that lies on top of our genes and influences whether they are modified, switched on, or switched off.[45]

You can see the impact of epigenetics in the way a queen bee and her worker bees look different and perform quite different functions. All the bees in a hive share the same DNA, but their genes are expressed differently.[46,47] The varied environments twins are exposed to can change their genetic expression so that their health is radically different over time. In your own life, genes that were switched off earlier may now be switched on, thanks to your lifestyle choices and the things you've been exposed to over the years.

2. Microbial Persistence

Microbial persistence allows the body to act in stealth mode. The infection secretes a protective shield called *biofilm* that effectively hides it from the immune system. This prevents antibiotics from getting to it. Since bacteria cannot get the nutrients they need to grow, they slow down and may even go into hibernation.[3] Without dynamic bacteria to combat, any antibiotics we use against the bacteria are likely to be completely ineffective.

Borrelia burgdorferi, the bacteria that causes Lyme disease, is known to secrete biofilms when it is under stress (such as when we are trying to kill it with antibiotics). Scientists now suspect that this may be one reason Lyme disease can be so difficult to eradicate.[48]

When an infection is hidden in a biofilm, the acquired immune system recognizes that there is a persistent infection in our body, but it can't kill it because it can't get near it. This exasperating situation drives our immune system a bit crazy. It ends up sending in antibodies anywhere it can – not only against the infection but also against our own tissue.

It's like an enraged dog attached to a leash that is too short to get at the cat that sits quietly, licking its paws, just out of range.

The National Institutes of Health reports that 80 percent of infections associated with chronic disease are associated with biofilm formation.[49] Knowing this is crucial to our strategy. In order to eradicate chronic infections, we need to develop agents that help break up the biofilms, so we can find the persistent microbial infections they hide. We can also employ medications that are able to penetrate the biofilm and kill the infections underneath.

3. Bystander Activation

Bystander activation occurs when other immune cells get into the fight they were not originally involved in because the immune system is hyper-reactive. They start attacking not only the infection but also healthy tissues that should have remained out of the brawl.

It's like a honky-tonk bar where everyone's a bit drunk and judgment is not at its finest. John is upset by Bill making a pass at his girlfriend. Words are exchanged, tempers quickly flare, and fisticuffs ensue. John hits Bill. Bill falls back and knocks a pitcher of beer onto Steve. Steve, who knows neither John nor Bill, believes Bill assaulted him and pushes him into George and... you get the idea.

Knowing about bystander activation allows us to understand inappropriate activation of the immune system.

Infections can trigger one or all of these mechanisms in the body and result in autoimmunity.

The rule is simple: If you don't look, you will not find. If there is an infection in your body, it needs to be eliminated, and the damage it has caused to your immune system needs to be addressed too. If either one of these steps is missing, you will not heal.

HOW AUTOIMMUNITY BEGINS

After returning from his honeymoon in the Caribbean, Chad, a 26-year-old athlete in excellent health, felt an inexplicable pain in his right ankle. No trauma, no swelling, just pain. By evening, he was suffering from chills and sweats. Then, to make things a little more interesting, a strange bout of muscle twitches started.

His family physician initially did blood work and tested him for a viral infection, but his tests were normal. The fever and chills only lasted a week, but the ankle pain and muscle twitching did not let up.

At his doctor's suggestion, he went to a podiatrist who could not find the cause of the ankle pain, and a neurologist, who declared that Chad's nerve tests, MRI, and blood work were all normal.

In a few months, when the ankle pain subsided, Chad felt better, but not quite back to normal. Over the next year, he fought a low-grade fatigue that got progressively worse. At first, he noticed his workouts were a little tougher. When he developed neck and shoulder pain, chiropractic adjustments helped, but only temporarily. Over time, simple things like trying to carry groceries were exhausting. When his son was born a year later, his right arm was too painful and too weak to hold his new baby boy.

This time, an MRI showed a small, herniated disc in his neck pressing on the nerve to his right arm. The neurologist referred Chad to a physical therapist. The therapy helped alleviate the neck and shoulder pain, but the fatigue continued to progress.

When Chad developed a tremor in his hands, the neurological tests again came back normal. When he developed an irregular heartbeat and shortness of breath, the cardiology tests were normal too.

All of his treatments were workarounds. The doctors and specialists were looking at his body in pieces, as if its systems were isolated and mechanical, not interactive and organic. Since the main problem was being completely ignored, Chad's symptoms inevitably got much worse.

When I first met Chad, he had been struggling with progressively declining health for six years with no good explanation.

While he was still able to work, he rated his energy at 4 on a 10-point scale. He could no longer exercise. The slightest exertion gave him irregular heartbeats and shortness of breath. The muscle and joint pain that moved around his body, through his neck and shoulders, remained the worst issue he faced. But that's only because he had come to accept his constant fatigue, brain fog, inability to concentrate, and sensitivity to light. He consistently slept eight hours but never felt rested, and his sheets were always drenched from night sweats.

You might be surprised to hear that there are not a lot of things that can cause painful joints that move around the body intermittently. But Lyme disease is notorious for that. So, it became one of my top concerns. The night sweats left me concerned about babesiosis, a parasite infection transmitted by ticks.

An autoimmune process set off by these infections could cause the irregular heartbeat as well as many of the neurologic symptoms.

When the testing came back, we found that Chad had both Lyme and Babesia. He also had chronic Epstein-Barr. Not surprisingly, his vitamin D level was very low. Vitamin D is essential for a healthy functioning immune system. Chad also had clear markers for autoimmunity.

INFECTIONS THAT TRIGGER AUTOIMMUNITY

Unfortunately, missed infections are fairly commonplace in medicine. The five I find most frequently in the patients I see are all diseases you can get from enjoying being outdoors:

1. Lyme
2. Bartonella
3. Babesia
4. Chronic Epstein-Barr virus
5. Mycoplasma pneumonia

Tick bites infect more people in the Unites States with a disease every year than any other vector-borne infection. Vector is another name for the middleman that gives us the infection, typically a blood-feeding tick or insect, such as a mosquito or flea. Lyme disease, Zika virus, West Nile virus, and malaria are all vector-borne infections.

1.Lyme

In the United States, there are over 300,000 new cases of Lyme disease a year. It is the number one vector-borne infection.[50] Not all ticks carry Lyme disease, but the two that transmit the disease in the United States are the deer ticks: *Ixodes scapularis* in the northeastern, mid-Atlantic regions and *Ixodes pacificus* in the west.[51] The bug that causes the main two types of Lyme disease is *Borrelia burgdorferi*. It accounts for more than two-thirds of vector-borne diseases in the country.[5] In Europe and Asia, Lyme is caused by two different species, *Borrelia afzelii* and *Borrelia garinii*.[52,53]

The good news is that the treatment for all these different causes of Lyme is pretty much the same. One of the reasons the infection is often missed, however, is that doctors do not know to test for all the different species. We will discuss this issue more in the chapter on infectious diseases.

Lyme has been referred to as The Great Imitator. It can present with many different symptoms.

When it causes a fever, headache, rash, sweats, chills, and joint or muscle pain, doctors can easily assume it's the flu. It's commonly mistaken for chronic fatigue syndrome or fibromyalgia. Notoriously, Lyme is misinterpreted by doctors as mood and behavior disorders (ADHD, bipolar and monopolar depression) Parkinson's disease, Alzheimer's, and multiple sclerosis.[54][55][56]

Regardless of what the mistaken identity may be, Lyme disease is extremely dangerous if left untreated. It can damage the heart or nervous system. It can cause autoimmune nerve damage, causing loss of feeling and weakness in the legs and arms, as well as difficulty with focus, concentration, memory, and sleep disturbances, which can be quite severe. (One of my patients developed such severe insomnia that she was only sleeping three to four hours every few days.) Lyme disease has been linked to the onset of pediatric acute-onset neuropsychiatric syndrome (PANS).[57]

As if Lyme disease wasn't bad enough, my Lyme patients often have other infections to go with it, because the tick that transmits Lyme disease can also carry a number of other infections, such as *Anaplasma, Ehrlichia, Bartonella, Babesia,* and the recently identified *toxoplasmosis.*[58]

Anaplasma and Ehrlichia respond to the treatments we use for Lyme, but should be tested for, identified, and tracked until it is eradicated. Bartonella and Babesia require a different treatment, so it is critical to test for them any time Lyme is present. One study reported a 78 percent occurrence of a co-infection with Bartonella in a group of chronic Lyme patients.[59] Other studies have found that 20 to 50 percent of the ticks that carry Lyme also carry Babesia.[60]

Mononucleosis is another common co-infection of Lyme.

2. Bartonella

Bartonella can be caused by bites from fleas and body lice, as well as ticks. There are, of course, several species of Bartonella. Why make this easy? The one we are mainly concerned about here is Bartonella henselae. Some Bartonella symptoms overlap with Lyme, but there are differences – visual problems, anxiety, and depressive symptoms particularly resistant to treatment, lymph node enlargement, and a variety of neurologic disorders including seizures. A particularly distinctive symptom of Bartonella is the development of a skin rash that looks like stretch marks that have a red or purple color to them. The rash can be quite dramatic.

One of my patients developed bold red stria across the middle of his back. The dermatologist agreed that it was a Bartonella rash, but the infectious disease specialist told my patient and his mother that the rashes where the result of "cutting behavior." We were dumbfounded that this physician would actually accuse my patient of intentionally harming himself by cutting his skin to create the rash, especially when the rash was in the middle of his back in an area he could barely reach, not to mention the fact that there was absolutely no evidence of the skin being cut.

3. Babesia

This parasite causes a disease called Babesiosis that is transmitted by a tick and can look very much like malaria. If you have a Babesia infection with a Lyme infection, it will basically make all of the symptoms you have worse – fevers, fatigue, chills, day and night sweats, and in some it will cause an unexplained cough or a sense of air hunger. Air hunger is this sense that even though your lungs are fine, you do not feel like you are getting enough air when you breathe. There may be some changes in the blood work, but what you need to make this diagnosis is what we call in medicine "a high index of suspicion." That's a fancy phrase for saying you have to have thought this might be the problem or at least part of the problem and then run the proper testing.

4. Chronic Epstein-Barr Virus

Mononucleosis, also known as mono or sometimes the Rip Van Winkle Bug, is caused by the Epstein-Barr Virus (EBV). It is an infection almost all of us have had in childhood or adolescence. Also called the kissing disease, when acute, it causes swollen lymph nodes, fever, and fatigue, which can be quite severe. The infection can also cause the liver and spleen to swell. Remember that friend in high school who got sick and was given permission by their physician to sleep for 12–14 hours a day? How about the kid who got sick and needed to stop playing sports for a month or so because their spleen was swollen? These were your friends who had mono.

For most of us, mono was either a mild infection or one we completely recovered from within a few weeks. For all of us who have had mono, the virus lies latent in us, not causing any problems, but still in our system. When our immune system gets suppressed, such as when we get Lyme disease or from toxic exposure, the EBV can reactivate, making us sick.

Think about shingles. It is caused by a chicken pox virus (a relative of EBV, by the way) that continued to live inactive in a kind of suspended animation (think Han Solo in carbonite) in one of our nerve roots near the spine. It cannot go anywhere because our immune system will not let it. One day our immune system gets distracted by another infection (various tick-borne diseases), a toxic exposure (heavy metals, mold toxins, herbicides), or a medication that suppresses our immune system (steroids), and the chickenpox virus escapes, crawls out along the nerve into the area of our skin that the nerve provides sensation to, and now erupts onto the skin as a painful rash.

In the exact same way that the chicken pox virus can reemerge, its sibling EBV can also get reactivated when our immune system gets distracted. Reactivated EBV has been linked to some cases of chronic fatigue syndrome (ME/CFS), and there is research that suggests a possible link to fibromyalgia, through the research here is very preliminary.[61,62] Acute EBV infection has also been linked to the onset of PANS.

5. Mycoplasma Pneumonia

This infection shows up in people whose immune systems are already compromised. Its presence activates the acquired immune system and can trigger autoimmunity.

This invasive pest is a part of a group of bacteria that lack a true cell wall. Instead, they are held together by a membrane. Since antibiotics like penicillin work by attacking the cell wall, they will not work against mycoplasmas.

The most famous member of this family is mycoplasma pneumonia (M. pneumonia). It is often called atypical or "walking pneumonia" where you look and feel a whole lot better than your chest x-ray suggests you should feel. Many of us have had a mild form of mycoplasma pneumonia, but since immunity doesn't last, it frequently returns later to make us sicker and more resistant to treatment.[63] Other members of the family are M. hominis, M. felis, M. arginine, and M. salivarium. The mycoplasmas have also been linked to chronic asthma, bronchitis, joint pain, and autoimmune diseases, such as Crohn's disease, rheumatoid arthritis, PANS and ME/CFS. [64, 65]

The range of symptoms associated with mycoplasma infections is somewhat intimidating for those of us who need to remember these things. They can involve virtually the entire body. People with a mycoplasma can suffer with severe fatigue, muscle pains, joint pains, eye problems, heart problems, lung problems, digestive disorders, liver disease, neurologic disorders, such as brain inflammation (encephalitis), meningitis, and the list goes on.

With a hidden infection, your entire immune system has been undermined. The problem is frequently multilayered with multiple infections occurring at the same time. Treatment requires first identifying all of the infections present, then eliminating them.

The infections I've mentioned in this chapter are by no means an exhaustive list, but a list of those infections that are most commonly missed. It is the responsibility of your physician to test and treat appropriately. It is when these infections remain hidden that you get even sicker because you develop autoimmunity, and your own immune system starts to attack you.

PART II

WHAT SETS YOU UP FOR AUTOIMMUNE DISEASE?

Ideally, when an infection hits, your immune system will respond with the efficiency for which it is renowned. You will be sick for a while, then bounce back as healthy as ever. But if you are suffering from autoimmunity, that's not what happens.

At some point, you got an infection. That infection may have been impossible to shake, or it may have seemed to fade, simmering in the background, draining the best resources of your health. In Part I, we learned that Step 1 is to eliminate the infection once and for all.

Step 2 is to find out what set you up for an autoimmune response in the first place. The four most common culprits are:

- **Unhealthy Sleep:** Losing even one night's sleep impairs your ability to fight off infections and reduces the potency of vaccines against infection by 50 percent.
- **Abused Gut:** An imbalanced gut increases the odds of autoimmune disease.
- **Environmental Toxins:** Pollution can damage the immune systems of unborn children and their children for generations.
- **Emotional Trauma:** People with stress disorders, like PTSD, are far more likely to develop autoimmune diseases.

When your body is already set up for a fall with poor sleep, gut imbalance, toxins, and trauma, an infection can easily be the final assault that overwhelms your struggling immune system and makes it give way to autoimmune disease.

CHAPTER 4

—

UNHEALTHY SLEEP

- *The top four sleep issues that impair health*
- *How too little sleep can make you vulnerable to infection*
- *How a few days of poor sleep impact your heart, your hormones, and your insulin balance*

Sleep issues are the number one problem among my patients. Virtually all of my patients struggle with sleep, but the nature of one patient's struggle is often radically different from that of another.

Barbara can't go to sleep. It's not uncommon for her to sleep on Monday from 7:00 a.m. till 9:00 a.m., then not sleep again till Thursday afternoon from 3:00 p.m. till midnight. Anna Marie, by contrast, is the queen of sleep. On the nights when she manages to get to bed by 10:00 p.m., she's up at crack of noon for a quick bite to eat before falling back to sleep on the couch until dinnertime. Some days, she sleeps 18 hours a day.

For both Barbara and Anna Marie, sleep issues are their secondary diagnosis. One sleeps too little, the other sleeps too much, yet they share an underlying problem: their immune systems are in hyper-drive, causing brain inflammation.

Sleep issues that result from brain inflammation are especially complicated. First, we have to figure out whether your sleep problem is a primary or a secondary problem. We have to ask ourselves: Is your sleep causing your other complaints or are your other complaints affecting your sleep?

When sleep is your primary problem, your brain becomes inflamed because poor sleep is causing your immune system to malfunction. If sleep is your secondary problem, something has activated your immune system and inflamed your brain, which then resulted in poor sleep.

To resolve the problem, we take the same steps you've read about in the preceding chapter. First, we learn what set the fire in the brain, then we eliminate those conditions, then we put out the smoldering inflammation that remains in the immune system.

WHAT IS SLEEP?

Sleep is a dynamic activity. In America, we thought of sleep as a passive, dormant part of our lives until the 1950s. Now we realize that our brains are very active during sleep.

We're still trying to understand all the ways in which sleep is essential to us, but what we do know is that, without the vital activities going on while we sleep, our ability to function as well as our physical and mental health are quickly impaired.[66]

Sleep is a complex event necessary for health and healing. It detoxifies your brain, keeping you healthy and sane. Our most exciting discoveries about brain detoxification have only happened recently.

We've long known that the entire body – except the brain – has a delicate waste removal system called the lymphatic system. It gets rid of the garbage generated by our cells all day long, as well as toxins from the environment. A crucial component of the immune system, the lymphatic system is the body's garbage disposal workforce and police force combined.

For a long time, as far as we knew, the brain had no way to manage its own waste and dispose of toxins. Then, in 2015, Dr. Antoine Louveau and his team at the University of Virginia discovered lymphatic connections from the brain to the rest of the body. This means we have to entirely reassess our understanding of how the immune system of the brain works![67]

Just three years earlier, Dr. Jeffrey Iliff and his team at Ohio State University found that the brain actually possesses its own unique form of a lymphatic system. They called it the *glymphatic system*. Particularly exciting was the discovery that the glymphatic system is active at night while we sleep.[68]

This confirms that the brain must remove accumulated waste and toxins just like the rest of the body. And it does so during sleep.

Healthy sleep has stages 1, 2, 3, 4, and REM (rapid eye movement). The stages are determined by the wave forms we see when we measure brain waves with an electroencephalogram (EEG). It is not a smooth progression from one stage to the next during the night. Instead, we move from stage 2 to REM sleep (the dream stage), then start over again. As much as 50 percent of our total sleep time stays in Stage 2. We spend 20 percent in REM sleep. The other 30 percent is spread out among Stages 1, 3, and 4. Almost all of our time asleep is spent in Stages 1, 2, and REM.[69]

REM is so essential, that if our REM sleep is disrupted one night, it changes the entire pattern. Instead of starting with Stage 1 the next night, we rush to catch up on our REM sleep first. Throughout that night and the next ones, we spend extended periods of time in REM until we catch up.[70]

If that doesn't tell you how important REM sleep is, consider this. Lab rats normally live for two to three years. But in studies cited by the American Sleep Association, lab rats deprived of REM sleep only survive for five weeks. If they are deprived of sleep altogether, they die in three weeks.[71]

Considering how disastrous it can be when we get too little sleep, it's strange that we often pride ourselves on functioning with less sleep. We are literally taking years off our lives and acting as if it were a virtue.

Today, about 33 percent of the population sleeps six or fewer hours per night. Only 33 percent sleeps eight hours or more. Yet loss of sleep slows brain metabolism by seven percent, resulting in performance deficits, poor physical and mental reaction time, increased errors, decreased vigilance, impaired memory, and reduced motivation.[72]

WHEN SLEEP GOES WRONG

Doctors have identified more than 70 sleep disorders. At least 40 million Americans each year suffer from some kind of chronic sleep disorder. Another 20 million suffer from occasional sleeping issues. Most issues can be managed effectively if they are correctly diagnosed.[73] If they are not treated, serious health issues can develop.

Sleep disturbances can be a tricky problem to address. We need to be very thoughtful in our approach to both identify the problem and find the cure. It is especially important that we understand the problem so we don't make things worse.

With less than six to eight hours of sleep, profound changes begin to take place in the endocrine, cardiovascular, and immune systems, and insulin resistance occurs. Restoring normal endocrine and immune function typically requires three days of nine-and-a-half or more hours of sleep. More time may be needed. Studies showing 8–14 hours of sleep a day for more than a month resulted in continuous improvement.[74]

Neurons in your brainstem connecting your brain to your spinal cord produce serotonin and norepinephrine to keep the brain active while you are awake. As you fall asleep, other neurons turn off the signals that have been keeping you awake.[75]

SLEEP AND YOUR IMMUNE SYSTEM

The immune system's main function is to defend us from infections caused by pathogens.

On the other hand, sleep has attracted particular interest lately for its potential impact on the immune system.[76]

It is thought that sleep actually modulates the immune system and, thereby, plays a vital role in fending off infection. Medical researchers are just beginning to explore the connection between sleep, infections, and their impact on the immune system. When an infection invades the body, numerous metabolic functions have to change in order to get rid of the pathogen.[77]

Sleep is essential to our immune response. Without it, our immunity is weakened, making us more vulnerable to viral, bacterial, and parasitic infections. Numerous studies show that deprivation of REM sleep alters the immune system, changing neurotransmitters, hormones, and cytokines. There seems to be mutual adjustment between our sleep and our immune system by means of a constant two-way communication.

We know that infections often change sleep patterns, but we do not understand exactly why that happens. Viruses such as Covid-19, influenza, and immunodeficiency virus (HIV) are often characterized by fever, fatigue, and altered sleep patterns. Bacterial infections can also produce changes in sleep, such as narcolepsy and insomnia. Studies in animals show sleep disturbances associated with Lyme disease caused by *Borrelia burgdorferi*, rhombencephalitis caused by *Listeria*, bacterial meningitis, sarcoidosis, and pneumococcal meningitis.[78]

Among patients with narcolepsy, a large percentage have antibodies to bacterial infections such as *Streptococ-*

cus and *Helicobacter pylori*. It raises the question as to whether sleep disorders like narcolepsy may be triggered by autoimmune mechanisms.[79]

In order to find out, researchers conducted a study to see if sleep could protect the body against infection by parasites. In 12 different species of mammals, they found that the longer the animals slept, the less likely they were to have a parasitic infection.[80]

The impact of sleep on our immune system is profound. Studies show that missing a night's sleep reduces the effectiveness of vaccines by 50 percent.[81] After being exposed to a virus, you are far more likely to get sick if you are chronically sleep-deprived. Because your body function is impaired, it will also take significantly longer to recover.

Cytokines and antibodies that fight infections and inflammation are released by the immune system during sleep. If sleep is impaired, the body has fewer solutions for fighting off infection. Chronic sleep deprivation or poor sleep has repeatedly been shown to heighten the risk of diabetes, obesity, and cardiovascular disease.[82]

If adults get too little sleep (less than six hours) or too much sleep (more than nine hours), it confers a higher risk for the development of autoimmune diseases such as RA, SLE, and Sjogren's. It sets off a vicious cycle. The autoimmune disorders make brain inflammation worse, which makes sleep worse, which makes the autoimmune disorder worse.[83]

The immune system has its own circadian rhythm, so *when* we sleep is also important. Different parts of the immune systems are active at different times of day. While we used to think that the body would adjust to widely varying sleep cycles, recent studies show that sleeping at night is crucial to the normal regulation of both the innate and the adaptive immune systems.[84]

Too little sleep makes us more prone to infection. Losing even four or five hours impairs the ability of the natural killer cells in your immune system to fight off viral infections and cancer.[85] As you might imagine, getting too little or too much sleep on a regular basis increases our risk of getting colds, or even pneumonia.[86]

Endocrine Effects

Not getting enough sleep for just *four days* will make your thyroid hormone levels rise.

Growth hormone, which is released during slow-wave brain activity in the deep stages of sleep, regenerates tissues, the immune system, and lean body mass. If those hours of sleep are interrupted, you may suffer the effects of too little growth hormone: depression, weight gain, reduced muscle mass, and insulin resistance.[87]

Heart Attacks

Getting less than five hours of sleep a night for two or more days a week resulted in a 200 to 300 percent increase in heart attacks in men in one study. (That is five to ten times the risk of having high cholesterol.) In women, it resulted in an 82 percent increase.[88]

Insulin Resistance

In one study, the body's ability to clear glucose was depressed by 40 percent after test subjects slept four hours a night for four days.[89] Eating carbohydrates within three hours of sleep creates an insulin response that blocks growth hormone production too. Valium, Xanax, and other medications block the surge of growth hormone by preventing deep sleep altogether.[90]

Getting less sleep than your body needs runs up a "sleep debt." You will pay for it in impaired judgment, lower reaction time, and greater sensitivity to pain, as well as:

- Weakened immune system
- Weight gain
- Colds, flu, pneumonia
- Depression
- Increased risk for heart disease
- Increased risk for Type 2 diabetes
- Reduced life span

Poor sleep can lead to immune dysfunction and brain inflammation, or brain inflammation can lead to poor sleep. In either event, it is a very serious problem that we need to address.

YOUR SLEEP

The average adult needs seven to nine hours of sleep a night to be healthy. Teenagers need between nine to ten hours a night for optimal health. Normally, it should take you less than 30 minutes to fall asleep. You may awaken briefly once or twice, but otherwise, you should sleep soundly through the night. When you awaken in the morning you should feel refreshed.

There is a Goldilocks effect – too much is bad or too little is bad, and just right is what you need. What this means is that poor health is associated with both consistently getting too little sleep (less than six hours) and too much sleep (more than ten hours).

To evaluate your sleep, let's start with a quick sleep history I use with all my patients:

1. What time do you go to bed?
2. Do you take anything to help you get to sleep? If so, what?
3. How long does it take you to fall asleep?
4. Do you have trouble falling asleep? If so, why (for

example, your mind filled with worries, your arms or legs feel uncomfortable and need to move, your body is in pain)?

5. Do you sleep through the night, or do you wake up in the middle of the night? If so, what wakes you up? How long do you stay awake? How many times a night?
6. Do you snore?
7. Has anyone noticed you struggling to breathe or stop breathing during sleep?
8. What time do you awaken to start your day?
9. How often do you feel rested?
10. Do you need to take naps? How many times a day or week? How long?

Sleep questionnaires like this can only give us a general impression, since most of us are not very good at accurately reporting on the amount and quality of our sleep. Fortunately, there are a number of devices that help us get a better understanding of what's actually going on.

Most activity trackers can track the number of hours you sleep, the number of times you wake up, and the duration of time you're awake. One of the newest devices on the market is the Oura ring. Since I am not a fan of watches myself, I particularly like the Oura ring (https://ouraring.com). Although it is not an FDA-approved device, I have checked the sleep results reported by the Oura ring against the results of an FDA-approved sleep monitoring device and I am impressed with the ring's accuracy.

Activity trackers are invaluable in helping me objectively quantify my patients' sleep patterns so I can monitor their recovery. Their data is also helpful when I need to make an argument with the insurance company about the extent of my patients' disabilities.

TYPES OF POOR SLEEP

"A good night's sleep is when you fall asleep quite easily, do not fully wake up during the night, do not wake up too early, and feel refreshed in the morning. Regularly having difficulty falling asleep or sleeping through the night is not normal."[91]

The list of things that make sleeping difficult is a long one: a noisy neighborhood, an uncomfortable bed, someone snoring next to you, a baby crying in the other room, a mind preoccupied with events of the day, a work shift at odd hours, or a TV show so good you can't stop binge-watching it. Beyond that, medication, illness, stress, alcohol, drugs, or sleep apnea are common culprits, but bruxism (teeth grinding), somnambulism (sleep walking), nightmares, talking in your sleep, or jetlag can throw off your sleep cycle too. And almost half of us snore.[92]

When it comes to sleep, these are some of the most common complaints:

1. **Insomnia** is the top complaint. This year, like every other year, nearly 82 million Americans will experience insomnia. Fortunately, 75 percent of them will recover without developing persistent problems with sleep.[93]

2. **Sleep Apnea** is the most chronic issue, affecting as many as 22 million Americans.[94]

3. **Circadian Rhythm Sleep Disorders** cause problems for nearly ten million Americans, since they result from a misalignment of the body's internal biological clock. Without that internal regulation, it is very difficult to know when to go to sleep and when to wake up!

4. **Narcolepsy** only affects about 200,000 Americans, but it can result in very undesirable effects, such as sleep paralysis, cataplexy, and hallucinations.[95]

Insomnia

You may have trouble sleeping for a variety of reasons. Whether you fall asleep easily but wake up in the night and can't get back to sleep, or you can't fall asleep in the first place, we call it *insomnia.*

Poor sleep in any form can result in an inability to concentrate, depression, sleepiness, and lack of energy. Reaction time and learning decrease by 50 percent after only 17 to 19 hours without sleep. This means that working through the night is increasingly counterproductive. It's worth remembering that if you get up at 7:00 a.m. and are not asleep by midnight, your level of functioning is already seriously impaired.[96]

After just one day without sleep, your ability to function is worse than if you were legally drunk. Staying awake for 24 hours is like a blood-alcohol level of 0.10 percent. In the United States, 0.08 percent is the legal limit.[97]

The levels of severity for insomnia are *transient* (less than a week), *acute* (up to a month), and *chronic* (more than a month). Both transient and acute insomnia can be brought on by external stressors. A noisy neighborhood, a new job, financial worries, family pressures, or a new baby are just a few examples. When insomnia becomes chronic, medical and psychological issues should be explored.

Sleep Apnea

When breathing stops and starts in the night, it can be an indication of this serious sleep disorder. In some cases, when the throat muscles relax, they obstruct the airway (*obstructive sleep apnea*). When the brain sends the wrong signals to the muscles that control breathing, it can cause *central sleep apnea*. If a combination of both issues occurs, we refer to it as *complex sleep apnea syndrome.*

Loud snoring is not necessarily a sign of sleep apnea, but it can be. Snoring can be caused by or result in very poor breathing that starves your brain of oxygen and annoys your sleeping companions. Not everyone with sleep apnea snores, but if there were an Olympic event in snoring, I would win the gold. All my life, I'd been a high-energy, motivated, around-the-clock kind of guy, who swam a few miles a week, stayed up doing research till 1:00 a.m., and snored loudly enough at night to blow the doors off. My wife and I slept at the far end of our five-bedroom house. And still the kids complained!

Apart from the jokes at my expense and the loss of sleep on everybody else's, I assumed it was just a laughable quirk. And then I started getting lots of colds and at least one major bout of pneumonia every year. Over time, I needed more and more sleep. When I woke up in the mornings, I didn't feel rested at all. I reluctantly went in for a sleep study at Georgetown, but the sleep study was normal. There was no evidence of sleep apnea. This was in the very early days of understanding the diagnosis of sleep apnea.

Over the next few years, things got progressively worse. One of the issues I was having was terrible acid reflux. An exam by the gastroenterologist confirmed the reflux problem, but my doctor didn't see a pattern and recommended antacids.

My wife Fran, who is a lawyer though claims she was a physician in a past life (actually she might have been. She is a frighteningly good diagnostician at times.), insisted the first sleep study was wrong. "You have sleep apnea," Fran said.

Indeed, I was exhausted all the time. I would sleep nine hours and feel like I hadn't slept at all. I started falling asleep everywhere: in the movies, at stop signs, riding in the car as a passenger. I struggled to stay awake while doing things that interested me, like spending time with my family or interviewing patients.

"You have to get another test," Fran said. "You stop breathing at night."

So, I went in for another study. This time, the sleep apnea results were bad – worse than anyone I'd ever diagnosed!

My Apnea Index was 42 (less than five is normal). Oxygen saturation in the blood should be 94–96. Untreated, mine dropped as low as 64. I was having 236 apneas an hour (219 obstructive and 19 central). If I kept this up, I'd be dead soon.

With that diagnosis, I started using the CPAP (continuous positive airway pressure) machine all night, every night. Within a week, my energy was completely back. I was feeling rested after seven hours of sleep. I've had no further incidents of bronchitis or pneumonia since. In a year, the reflux had disappeared. And, to the relief of my entire family, I finally stopped snoring.

I had been well on my way to a heart attack. My sleep apnea was suppressing my immune system and causing acid reflux. Next, I would've gotten high blood pressure. With a significantly higher risk of heart disease, a heart attack would have only been a matter of time. Sleep apnea is a serious matter.

Sleep apnea affects five percent of us and about 85 percent of people with sleep apnea don't know they have it. Sleep apnea can affect children as well as adults. If you have sleep apnea, taking medications to help you sleep or for pain may dramatically worsen the sleep apnea. Untreated sleep apnea increases your risk for obesity, diabetes, hypertension, heart disease, and stroke. Sleep apnea significantly impairs the functioning of the immune system.[98] Studies increasingly demonstrate that untreated sleep apnea significantly raises the risk of developing autoimmune diseases.[99] Untreated sleep apnea can reduce your life expectancy by ten years.[100]

Think you might have sleep apnea? Take the Epworth test on my website, kaplanclinic.com/sleep-apnea/. If you score a ten or more, talk with your physician about further testing.

Circadian Rhythm Sleep Disorders

All living organisms and, indeed, every physiological function, has sleep and wake cycles. We call it the circadian rhythm. In Latin *circa* means "approximately" and *diem* means "day." A disorder of this pervasive natural rhythm is known as a *circadian rhythm sleep disorder* (CRSD).

As with insomnia, CRSD may cause you to have trouble falling asleep or staying asleep. You may simply wake up too early and not be able to go back to sleep. Variations include:

- **Delayed Sleep Phase Disorder:** Consistently staying awake more than two hours later than the normal sleep-wake cycle is considered a disorder. Night owls can fall into this category. It is most common in adolescents or young adults who prefer to stay up late into the night.[101]

- **Advanced Sleep Phase Disorder:** Either falling asleep too early (6:00 to 9:00 p.m.) and/or waking up too early (2:00 to 5:00 a.m.) also qualifies as a disorder. In this case, it is more common in middle-aged or elderly adults.[102]

- **Irregular Sleep-Wake Rhythm Disorder:** Regular naps and erratic patterns of sleep fall under this disorder with an undefined sleep-wake cycle.[103] Polyphasic sleep is a deliberately induced form of irregular sleep-wake rhythm disorder. One of the most popular approaches is a 90-minute to six-hour "core" sleep with 20-minute naps throughout the day. Others train themselves to take 20-minute naps all day for a total of two to three hours of sleep. The idea is that since the body defaults to slow wave and REM sleep when it is deprived of sleep, little bursts of sleep will allow them to cut back on sleep and spend more productive hours awake.[104] Scientific evidence says otherwise.

- **Jet Lag Disorder:** Ordinary jet lag is a transient effect, but if you move through time zones often enough, it can disturb your body's internal clock enough to result in an ongoing disorder. As with any jet lag, the experience is more difficult when traveling east than west, because the body adjusts to a delay in sleep better than an advance in sleep.[105]

Circadian rhythm sleep disorders are often misdiagnosed, and this results in health complications. Until recently, we have had a limited number of practical tools to evaluate and measure individual circadian rhythms. Treatment has included melatonin or light, but their impact on CRSD has not been rigorously tested in multicenter randomized clinical trials.[106]

The good news is that NIH studies have begun to show remarkable "…advances in our understanding of the molecular, cellular and physiological mechanisms underlying the regulation of circadian rhythms, as well as the impact of circadian dysfunction on health and disease." Soon we may have entirely new methods for treating CRSD.[107]

Narcolepsy

The word *narcolepsy* comes from two Greek words (*narkē lepsis*) meaning "seized by sleepiness."[108] "Narcolepsy is a chronic neurologic disorder that affects the brain's ability to control sleep-wake cycles."[109] While the condition is relatively rare, affecting about one in every 2,000 people, there is a significant overlap in the symptoms of ME/CFS, chronic depression, and chronic fatigue associated with other diseases. Also, people with narcolepsy have ten times more traffic accidents, so it's a problem you don't want to miss.[110]

People with narcolepsy struggle with excessive daytime sleepiness not relieved by sleep, brain fog (a problem with focus, concentration, and short-term memory), as well as disrupted sleep. As with many sleep disorders, a number of my patients suffer from narcolepsy and other medical conditions, such as post-treatment Lyme syndrome, fibromyalgia, depression, and ME/CFS.

There is increasing evidence that narcolepsy is the result of an autoimmune disorder, possibly one set off by the flu.[111]

It is important to identify each layer of the problem like peeling an onion, so we can treat all of the issues. Missing one will leave you still sick and suffering. What's worse, driving with narcolepsy can become life-threatening. With cataplexy, even walking down a flight of stairs can put you at risk for injury or death.

There are five primary symptoms of narcolepsy, identified by the acronym **CHESS**.

C Cataplexy occurs with a brief loss of muscle control causing you to collapse.

H Hallucinations may emerge as vivid dream-like experiences (hypnagogic hallucinations) as you fall asleep or as you wake up (hypnopompic hallucinations).

E Excessive daytime sleepiness can result in "sleep attacks."

S Sleep paralysis is the inability to move or speak during the transition between sleeping and waking.

S Sleep disruptions which involve frequently waking in the night.

For a quiz ranking your symptoms and likelihood of having narcolepsy, go to narcolepsylink.com.

As you can imagine, it's easy to mistake narcolepsy for something more common. Doctors estimate that it is misdiagnosed about 50 percent of the time.[112] For a conclusive diagnosis, you need to be evaluated by a sleep specialist.

All four of these disorders may occur along with other problems you are suffering from and make those problems much worse. They are especially important to catch, because fixing them may dramatically improve your condition, and missing them may prove life-threatening. Whatever type of poor sleep you experience, it has to improve for you to heal.

CHAPTER 5

—

ABUSED GUT

- *All disease begins in the gut.*
- *Our bodies are a vast ecosystem that has to stay in balance, or it breaks down.*
- *Chronic brain inflammation due to an impaired immune system is a growing epidemic.*

Sitting on a plane enroute to a conference in San Diego, I took another sip of coffee. I had booked back-to-back medical conferences and had gotten up late, so I'd had to grab a cup of coffee and a chocolate croissant at the airport for breakfast. It was not even vaguely a proper diet for me, but I told myself it was okay because I was in a hurry.

On the plane, my "lunch" included a roll and Asian chicken noodle salad. Lots of carbs, a little protein – all of it way too processed. When I settled down to get some work done, I was sound asleep after reading three pages, despite having a good night's sleep and waking refreshed just four hours earlier.

I had effectively poisoned myself. Specifically, I'd poisoned my second brain, the gut. When I did, it shut me down (I assume to prevent me from doing further damage to myself. My bad.)

You can't have a healthy brain if you don't have a healthy gut.

Every talk show, wellness book, and health guru in the last few years has talked about the gut, yet we still know relatively little about it. For centuries, it was dismissed as a kind of sewage system. It is so much more. The gut is the biggest immune system organ in our bodies.

For centuries, we've assumed that human beings were individual, self-determined organisms. As it turns out, we were wrong. We are symbiotic creatures. We could not live without the trillions of micro-organisms that populate our guts and outnumber our human DNA. These healthy flora:

- Protect against infections
- Modulate the immune process
- Regulate metabolism
- Digest food
- Make vitamins
- Manage the central nervous system
- Affect memory and emotions
- Produce 90 percent of serotonin in the body
- Promote cognitive function
- Support the blood-brain barrier
- Protect against invasion of organisms and toxins
- Prevent loss of electrolytes and water
- Allow absorption of fluids and nutrients

An unhealthy gut is associated with anxiety, depression, autism spectrum disorder, and allergies, as well as unconventional autoimmunity. We can make it worse with:

- Stress: physical or psychological
- Medications: NSAIDS, opioids, antibiotics, etc.
- Diet: high fat, high sugar, high fructose, gluten, alcohol
- Toxins: pesticides, BPA from plastics, mold
- Infections: viruses, bacteria, parasites

If we had any real grasp of how important it is to our health, we would never abuse it as casually as we do. In fact, the gut contains 70 percent of our immune system. It directly determines the health of every cell in our body – not only our immune system, but also our endocrine system and our brain.

WHAT'S IN THE GUT?

More than 2400 years ago, Hippocrates knew, "All disease begins in the gut." Today, science tells us that when it comes to gut bacteria, there are more of them than us: 150 trillion bacteria, 50 times the amount of human DNA in the body. What does that mean? We have a swarm of organisms living inside us that are vital to our existence.

Our second brain is not only made up of a massive assortment of bacteria, but also a multitude of other organism, viruses, and molds. These creatures in our stomach, small intestines, and large intestine collectively make up our gut microbiome. In all it weighs about four pounds (one-and-a-half times more than the brain in our skulls). Our microbiome is as unique to each of us as our own fingerprints.[113]

THE GUT AND AUTOIMMUNITY

In 2020, researchers around the world found that the risk of getting a severe Covid-19 infection was greatly increased with conditions that are associated with an imbalance of the gut microbiome, such as diabetes, high blood pressure, and obesity. The possibility that the gut microbiome may be able to predict the severity of Covid-19 prompted a flurry of additional research.[114]

We already know that the gut regulates our defenses against infections by activating the immune system's antiviral mechanisms and preventing inflammation. The gut has always played a crucial part in protecting us from infectious diseases, as well as gastrointestinal cancers, metabolic diseases, liver diseases, respiratory diseases, psychological diseases, and autoimmune diseases.[115]

We rely on our microbiome to protect us against infections, modulate our immune system, digest our food, make our vitamins, regulate our brain function, support our memory, and modulate our level of alertness. It helps determine how fast our food moves through our digestive tract and directly affects our resilience to stress.

The gatekeeper inside the gut is the intestinal wall. It doesn't often get the appreciation it deserves because it is basically a tube that runs through us. The inside of the intestine is like the outside of us, an extension of our skin, and it's the barrier between the interior and exterior world. Its job is to determine which substances we eat are going to be allowed into our bloodstream. If it fails, not only do toxins get through, but the components of ordinary food that should never be in our blood can also become dangerous. When that happens, we have "leaky gut."

The choices of the intestinal wall determine the quality of the nutrients that feed our cells. The proteins, neurotransmitters, and chemical messengers created by the microbiome are allowed through to travel to our brains and help regulate its functions (the vagus nerve is an even more direct way for the gut to communicate with the brain.)

The gut microbiome directly impacts the health and development of the immune system starting at birth and throughout life. The loss of diversity and specific families of bacteria in the gut microbiome are associated with many autoimmune diseases, including Crohn's disease, rheumatoid arthritis, and multiple sclerosis.[116]

This is a complex and evolving story. A 2018 study by Yale University researchers found that when a specific bacterium "escaped" from the gut into the blood because of a leaky gut, these bacteria induced an autoimmunity in those who were genetically predisposed to it.[117] In this and other studies, the best protection against autoimmunity was a healthy gut.[118]

The gut wall is responsible for about 70 percent of our immune system. The interaction between the gut wall and the micro-organisms inside the gut determine the health of our immune system.[119] That's why when bacteria escape into the blood stream from the gut, they can cause an autoimmune response.

It was previously believed that it took two components to develop a conventional autoimmunity: (1) genetic susceptibility and (2) problems in the gut. Emerging research shows that an infection, trauma, or toxic exposure can also set it off. Our ability to investigate these effects has become much more sophisticated and comprehensive in recent years with exciting advances like metabolomics, DNA sequencing, proteomics, and artificial intelligence bioinformatics.[120]

Gut problems are like cocking a trigger for autoimmunity. If it is already disturbed, the immune system is primed and ready for an event (infection, trauma, toxin) to fire the gun.

HARMING OUR SECOND BRAIN

Chili dogs, Whoppers, potato chips, orange things that crunch and taste like cheese but have no nutritional value – we literally starve the gut microbiome of the nutrients it needs to do its job and wonder why we don't feel well.

It is not just the food we eat that impacts the gut microbiome but also medication, supplements – basically anything we put in our mouths.

The anti-inflammatory medication we take for our aches and pains can cause ulcers in the stomach and small intestines. Antibiotics treat a strep infection in your throat, while they wipe out bacteria in your gut. It can take the gut microbiome months to years to return to normal.[121] After an infection accompanied by diarrhea, it can take the gut microbiota a month or longer to recover.[122]

Opioid painkillers can cause constipation, which in itself changes the balance of bacteria. Even worse, morphine decreases our ability to tolerate stress and makes us more susceptible to infections, worsening the overall inflammation throughout the body.[123]

Environmental toxins, such as pesticides, weed killers, and heavy metals, all damage the gut microbiome. I have a dear friend who is a health nut. He is very attentive to getting enough exercise, diet, and sleep. He makes a habit of doing what we all should do to maintain the best health possible, but even he found himself with mercury toxicity from eating too much fish. To make matters worse, lead toxicity has been found in a great deal of the water supply in the United States.[124]

Many of my patients who cannot tolerate wheat in any form in the United States can eat it without any side effects when visiting Europe. While there a number of factors that may explain the difference, the liberal use of herbicides containing glyphosate (the active ingredient in Roundup) in the States has been linked to an increase of both the celiac disease and the gluten intolerance now experienced by five percent of Americans.[125] It makes you wonder how much "gluten intolerance" and other digestive disorders associated with the food we eat is really intolerance to the poisoning of our food supply by pesticides and weed killers.

Apart from chemical toxins, the stress of the early-life separation of children from their parents results in changes of the gut microbiome that impair the endocrine system and immune systems.[126] These changes in the gut microbiome and resultant leaky gut may be responsible for the higher incidents of depression and autoimmunity seen in abused children later in life.[127]

Initially, an imbalanced gut may show up as a combination of brain fog, fatigue, chronic pain, headaches, sleep issues, and depression. Most doctors will not ask the right questions or do the right tests.

When the standard medical tests come back normal, the doctors tend to dismiss the complaints as random, unrelated symptoms, when in fact they are major warning signs that the immune system is under siege and fighting hard to save us. Instead of ignoring the signs, we should be letting them alert us to the danger, so we can help our immune system eliminate the problem and restore us to vigorous good health.

HOW IT HAPPENS

For Melissa, it started innocently enough on a hiking trip in Sao Paulo with her husband, Jason. She was very careful to drink bottled water, but didn't think twice about rinsing off her toothbrush from the tap. Bacteria from the local water moved into her gut, giving her a severe case of diarrhea.

Ordinarily "Montezuma's Revenge" is relatively easy to remedy, but Melissa couldn't shake it off. Her bowels, which had normally not been an issue for her, became irregular with bloating, gas, and episodes of cramping. About 13 percent of people who develop traveler's diarrhea go on to develop chronic irritable bowel syndrome (IBS).[128]

The bacterial infection disrupted the motility of her digestive tract and destroyed the normal balance of flora in Melissa's gut. Melissa's gut microbiome was now changed, and with it, her ability to digest certain foods, keep her gut wall healthy, and sustain her own health. This "reset" as a result of the infection and development of chronic IBS was not for the better. One of the consequences of this new "normal" was that Melissa's gut was now more permeable or leaky.

Remember that the health of our immune system and our brain is dependent on the gut, the gut wall, and the gut microbiome. The health of the gut wall relies on a delicate balance. It is the direct consequence of the food we eat, the health of the flora in the gut (our gut microbiome), and the motility of our digestive track.

Not everyone realizes that our food moves from our mouths because of a series of muscular motions starting with the tongue, moving down the esophagus to the stomach, and all the way through the digestive tract. Stress, infection, the food we eat, and gut microbiome imbalances can disrupt that motility. When the normal muscular contractions are impaired, the food gets sloshed back and forth instead of moving steadily in one direction.

When Melissa's healthy flora and the motility of the gut were disrupted, she began fermenting her food, resulting in gas and bloating. While this was socially and physically uncomfortable, it was only a symptom of the real problems that were brewing. In the state of imbalance of her gut microbiome, her gut wall became inflamed, permeable, and the gut barrier was disrupted.

But there was much more going on: A healthy gut microbiome is responsible for the production of vital nutrients such as multiple B vitamins and vitamin K. With the disruption of her gut microbiome, Melissa was also developing malnutrition of essential vitamins.[129] The gut microbiome also produces multiple signaling molecules, such as small chain fatty acids. Those signaling molecules are crucial to how the gut and brain communicate, as well as maintenance of brain health. When the gut-blood barrier is breached, the protective seal around the brain is disrupted as well. The gut microbiome impacts the structure and function of the brain. So, every function of the brain is affected. Melissa's brain health was being altered along with her gut microbiome, and not for the better.[130] The diarrhea in and of itself was also a problem, because with the excess fluid loss from the body, she was also losing magnesium in addition to other minerals.

Melissa's IBS symptoms were front and center. This was what had her attention and unfortunately the attention of her physicians. The focus was on the symptoms (diarrhea, bloating, and gas) and not the functions (brain health, vitamin production, immune health) of her gut. She was given medication to control the diarrhea. Melissa tried to explain to her doctor that she hadn't been able to concentrate very well since she got the infection, but he was focused on stopping the diarrhea and didn't consider it significant. The medications came with their own set of side effects – dry mouth, blurred vision. She attempted to alter her diet and over time noticed there were more and more foods that seemed to upset her stomach. Multiple visits to a variety of specialists resulted in variable improvements but no resolution of her problem. She has had good and bad periods, but over the years the IBS became her new normal.

Melissa had taken leave from her State Department job to do graduate studies at one of the top universities in the country. With the demands of her graduate program, Melissa was only now beginning to feel the real effects of brain inflammation set off by the IBS. Material that she used to master on the first reading now required several readings. Her writing started to lack the precision and clarity for which she had received accolades. She started drinking more coffee and caffeinated soda to compensate. At night, she tossed and turned, unable to get to sleep, and had to drag herself out of bed every morning.

As an adolescent, Melissa used to have inexplicable migraines several times a year. The migraines had lessened as she got older, but now they came roaring back. A neurologist prescribed Sumatriptan to constrict the blood vessels in her head. Since it can result in dizziness, muscle weakness, and nausea, she also gave Melissa Zofran, an anti-nausea medication that causes drowsiness. With every new symptom, the fire in her brain grew. The smoldering embers were building into a blaze. Melissa's health was being steadily undermined by the inflammatory process that started in her gut.

Despite all of the above – brain fog, fatigue, sleeplessness, migraines, IBS – Melissa soldiered on. She completed her graduate program, but not with the honors and accolades she was accustomed to. She and Jason returned to Washington where Melissa landed her dream job at the State Department.

The health of Melissa's brain and her immune system were dependent on the health of her gut wall and gut microbiome. Her risk for developing an autoimmunity had dramatically increased. The trigger was cocked, then disaster hit, and the gun went off.

It was February in D.C. and Melissa came down with what seemed like the flu. High fever, chills, headache, and a sore throat sent Melissa to bed utterly exhausted. Jason took her to urgent care where the physician checked her for strep throat and then agreed that this was probably flu. The next day she called her regular physician who agreed that it sounded like flu and recommended a prescription medication to help get over it faster. A week turned into two weeks and then the fever gradually went away, but the fatigue and exhaustion did not.

Sao Paulo was a distant memory. Three months after the "flu," Melissa went to her physician complaining of severe fatigue and sleep disturbances. Struggling at work, she had been feeling depression and having periods of anxiety. Her IBS was still an issue and something she had learned to live with. Her physical exam was "unremarkable", and when the standard labs tests came back normal, the diagnosis, of course, was the symptom not the disease, and she was referred to a psychiatrist for her "obvious" depression.

She had trouble tolerating the antidepressants, which caused dry mouth, worsening of her insomnia, and left her feeling totally flat emotionally with worsening of her fatigue. Where prior to the antidepressants she at least still had a good sex life with her husband, she was now unable to have an orgasm, which was less of a concern because she had also lost interest. Several antidepressants were tried, but frankly, "why bother" – they were certainly not making her feel better. The "depression" was manageable, and the medications just made her feel worse.

The treatment for her "depression" was not only ineffective, but she was also actually getting worse.

Over time the fatigue became crushing. She was sleeping 10–12 hours and never felt rested. Getting out of bed was a major event. Life became dragging herself through work and collapsing when she got home early in the evening. Housework and social events were a memory. Relatively minor activity put her in bed for days. She was told she had chronic fatigue syndrome.

THE GUT IN OUR ECOSYSTEM

As human beings, our health at any given moment reflects everything that's happened to us up till then – both physical and emotional. Nothing is isolated. Our bodies are like a jungle, a vast ecosystem where everything needs to stay in balance, or the entire system can break down.

That is why I start with a two-hour-long review of personal and medical history when someone like Melissa comes to my office. There are so many symptoms, so many layers of some-times conflicting medications, and all too often many, many years of suffering before they come to me.

I always ask: What was the tipping point? Was there a moment when you felt like yourself, then something hap-pened, and things have been going downhill ever since? Maybe you felt good for a few years, but another unexpected assault occurred, and all the old problems came rushing back?

When I take that history, I want to know everything that has the potential to contribute to the current wildfire in the brain. You can see why it takes so long. The standard practice of medical doctors allotting 15 minutes per patient just won't cut it. How can you hope to get to the root of the problem that fast? The best you can do is give the patient a stopgap, a drug to shut down the symptom, and send them on their way. I don't call that medicine.

To evaluate exactly what's going on with Melissa, I'd start with some common conventional testing and some specialized functional medicine testing of her blood, urine, and stool. The results will give us a place to start as we peel back the layers of inflammation.

Most likely, her tests would show a magnesium deficiency, leaky gut, and severe yeast overgrowth. Her magnesium defi-ciency isn't surprising, since both her imbalanced diet and her diarrhea deplete magnesium.

Because of her increasing sensitivity to food, she had started avoiding certain foods. Following the limitations of her doc-tor's recommended diet constricted the variety of her food even more. Soon she was hardly eating anything. She began to suf-fer from overall malnourishment.

The magnesium deficiency is an important one, but she was also losing a host of other vital nutrients. By cutting fats from her diet, her gut wall was becoming more permeable, since it needs small-chain fatty acids to support the gut lining. Melissa was not eating nuts, seeds, or leafy greens, which means her B vitamins were depleted. Too little magnesium made the receptors in her brain hypersensitive, which often results in migraines, fatigue, sleep disturbances, and other aches and pains.

Most Americans have low-levels of magnesium – partly because of the medications we take and partly because of the Standard American Diet (SAD). Think about it. Leafy greens, almonds, and beans are high in magnesium. Meat, milk, soda, and white flour are not. Common things such as coffee, tea, antacids, calcium supplements, birth control pills,[131] and sugar all deplete magnesium.[132] Alcohol doubles the excretion rate of magnesium.[133] As a result, most of us are in dire need of magnesium.

While we can often address the problem with an intravenous magnesium cocktail (a proprietary combination of high-dose vitamin C, B vitamins, magnesium and other vitamins) and dietary changes, in cases such as Melissa, magnesium levels are usually so low that it often takes as many as six to eight intravenous treatments to restore healthy magnesium levels to the body. Her yeast overgrowth could be treated with herbal supplements and diet. Acupuncture would be used to restore gut motility and also to reduce the inflammation in her brain. And low-dose naltrexone would reduce overall inflammation.

In three months, Melissa's headaches would be gone. In six months, her leaky gut would be dramatically better. We have gone a long way to restoring Melissa's health, but the exhaustion, depression, and anxiety remained significant issues.

That "flu" Melissa had a year earlier was not the flu. Melissa had developed mononucleosis. Almost everyone has had mono, a viral infection, and in most of us it is a relatively mild disease that we may have mistaken for a bad flu. Normally a self-limiting virus, it did not resolve in Melissa and was now chronic. Chronic mono is one of the bugs that has been linked to the development of ME/CFS. Other testing also reveals that Melissa was suffering with an autoimmunity that was attacking parts of her brain, most likely tripped off by the chronic mono.

The set-up was the IBS. Her dysfunctional gut impaired both her brain health but also her immune health. The gut issues showed up first with gas, bloating, cramping, irregular stools, and frequent diarrhea. The brain dysfunction with focus and concentration issues, low grade fatigue, and migraines was next. The rest of her immune system was also vulnerable, and when she developed mono, that was the final straw that set her own immune system against herself.

First, the doctors must quit chasing the symptoms and start addressing the problem: an inflamed leaky gut with gut microbiome dysbiosis and an inflamed brain (due to leaky gut, chronic mono, and autoimmunity).

So, the treatment is clear: fix and seal the gut, then address nutritional deficiencies caused by IBS, as well as the chronic mono infection and the autoimmunity.

The autoimmunity may resolve by healing her gut as above and resolving the chronic mono.

In some people, we need to go further. The next step will require working with a physician with advanced training in the use of specific medications, such as metformin, intravenous immunoglobin or Rituxan. Once the autoimmune issues are present, everything gets much more difficult to treat. But treatment and restoration to excellent health is possible.

It is a challenge, but within a year I would expect Melissa to be dramatically better.

MISTAKES TO AVOID

The symptoms are a distraction. Focusing on the root issues is the key. Melissa started out with traveler's diarrhea that resulted in what was diagnosed as chronic IBS. The problem evolved and her symptom list grew dramatically. Some of the symptoms caused by the medication given that were prescribed to help included:

- Diarrhea, bloating, and gas
- Multiple and growing food intolerances
- Fatigue
- Insomnia
- Brain fog and short-term memory loss
- Migraines
- Depression
- Anxiety
- Loss of interest in sex and unable to have orgasms
- Extreme exhaustion

Many people who start out with symptoms like Melissa's end up in nightmare scenarios. Occasional migraines turn into unremitting headaches, which are nearly unbearable and not responsive to treatment. Constant lack of sleep results in changes to personality and memory lapses that can cause poor job performance and loss of income. Inability to digest food, leaky gut, and irritable bowel syndrome lead to malnutrition and devastating conditions that can radically restrict mobility and leave you in constant pain. It becomes harder to socialize because of the exhaustion and depression. Marriages start to suffer because of constant physical problems, lack of libido, and disinterest in life. Sometimes patients lose their jobs or drop out of school and have to go on disability. The price for letting a fire rage in the gut that spreads to the brain and your immune system can be a horror story that none of us would want to live.

PEELING BACK THE LAYERS

For Melissa, several layers of symptoms overlapped. Her treatment was effective only because we removed each layer one by one. Once we seal the gut, the body will have the strength to join the fight to restore Melissa to health. We will have removed significant obstacles to its efforts by reducing inflammation and allowing it to absorb the nutrients it needs. Next, we will restore nutritional balance and sleep. Along the way, and as soon as possible, we will start removing the medications that are making things worse.

How she got to this state is obvious:

- **Infection:** "Montezuma's Revenge" from an infection changed the composition of the microbiome directly and indirectly changed the motility of her gut (leaky gut).
- **Antibiotics:** Antibiotics further disrupted the composition of the gut microbiome.
- **Extreme gut imbalance:** Ultimately, her leaky gut led to irritable bowel syndrome and inflamed her brain.
- **Proton Pump Inhibitors (PPIs):** Taking antacids and PPIs exacerbated the problems by changing the gut's pH balance.
- **Other medications:** Zoloft suppressed her orgasms and ability to get sound sleep. Bentyl blocked her symptoms without addressing the problems. Advil (ibuprofen) made her leaky gut worse (75 percent of people who take ibuprofen will develop ulcerations in the small intestines). Promethazine was only given to prevent the vomiting or nausea caused by other medications, so once we eliminate them, it is unnecessary. Sumatriptan and Dicyclomine can be eliminated immediately.
- **Sleep Disturbances:** When Melissa tells her doctors that she isn't sleeping well, they think of it as a symp-

tom they can medicate, not as a clue to the source of the problem. Brain inflammation interferes with sleep.

- **Depression**: With so many people taking antidepressants and complaining of depression, doctors are accustomed to writing a prescription. When they do, they miss an important part of the problem. They fail to connect the dots (depression is a symptom of an inflamed brain).

ONE EVOLVING PROBLEM, NOT MANY

When I look at Melissa, I don't see many problems; I see one problem that's evolving, cropping up in many different ways – just like a wildfire on the hillside igniting new shrubs.

Her gut is clearly not functioning. Her lack of sleep is creating inflammation by itself. I know that if we can reduce some of the inflammation – by getting her gut working again and restoring quality sleep – that will immediately help her migraines and diarrhea.

Removing the medications will eliminate a lot of symptoms too, but it's important to do it intelligently. Sometimes a patient can just stop taking medication, sometimes not. Medications were given for a symptom. It's ideal to treat the problem causing the symptoms first, then get rid of medication.

Throughout her treatment, I'm thinking about how I can address multiple things with diet, meditation, exercise, supplements, and, if necessary, medication that addresses the cause and not the symptoms. We do several things at once: heal and seal the gut, restore nutritional balance and deep sleep, and treat the chronic mono infection.

At this point, Melissa's symptoms should start to disappear. As they do, we can eliminate her medications one by one. In some cases, we can replace several strong medications with one gentler medication that addresses more problems. I'd put her on low-dose Amitriptyline or Pamelor, tricyclic antidepressants that would relax her gut, stop her diarrhea, and help alleviate both her headache and her depression. Ultimately, I would want to get her off all medications, but initially I'd look for medications that will do more with less. If we can replace several of Melissa's medication with one pill, it's a step in the right direction.

What we know for certain is that everything is interrelated. Having taken the time to ask questions and discover how these problems evolved, we are in a position to pick our battles.

The intravenous magnesium cocktail is crucial for correcting her malnourishment, so her body has the resources it needs to heal her. Acupuncture will help alleviate her inflammation and restore her gut balance. Manual therapy for her neck and upper back will help address her headaches.

I would explain to Melissa that her diet is making her significantly worse. Instead, I'd put her on a diet of rice, fish, chicken, fresh fruits, and vegetables. She has been drinking soda, which leaches much-needed calcium from her blood. To make matters worse, the soda is caffeinated, which irritates the gut, worsening the symptoms of IBS. A lot of her diet is based on pasta or bread made with white flour. A leaky gut is always more sensitive to gluten. Eliminating all gluten would help her enormously until we can seal the gut. If we don't seal the gut, the added nutrition we're giving her will leak out and keep her malnourished and inflamed.

A HIDDEN EPIDEMIC

In America, we are facing a growing epidemic of mysterious illnesses where some of the symptoms are treated – more or less effectively, often temporarily – and the others are dismissed by doctors as if they were unrelated. That leaves a smoldering fire of inflammation burning in the brain and impairs our immune system.

When the next assault comes along, it may seem fairly common – a bout of fever and chills in flu season, a hay fever attack that gets worse each spring, an acute attack of food poisoning, a whiplash injury from a minor car accident – but it will be mysteriously slow to heal. The body will not be as effective at tackling the problem, because it is still struggling to address old the fires in the gut and the brain that leave us trying to recover our health with an impaired immune system.

So, the flu, the allergies, the stomach upset, and the neck pain get worse. What should have been a fleeting assault becomes a chronic low-grade misery. The perpetual state of inflammation makes every new assault stick until the low-grade miseries add up to something worse. Instead of resolving, a case of the flu shows up as chronic fatigue, hay fever evolves into migraines, stomach upsets related to gut bacteria imbalance result in depression, or neck pain becomes fibromyalgia.

Our good health hinges on a paradox. Inflammation can provoke the most fatal diseases, yet it is vital to our survival. We need it to keep infections from festering, to heal abrasions, and to fight off toxins. Without inflammation, we die.

Oxygen is like that. Without it, our cells collapse. With too much of it, they collapse even faster.[134] Adrenaline keeps our blood pumping, but a sudden increase can stop our hearts.[135] Even drinking too many glasses of water can kill us.[136]

It's all about balance – a hard thing to sustain in our modern world where the potential for inflammation overload has grown exponentially. The worse culprits are the assaults that seem to go away but leave hidden inflammation behind.

Long after you believe you've let go of the heartbreak from a toxic relationship, the embers of inflammation from that trauma may be quietly burning. You were treated for Lyme disease, but never recovered. The cumulative effect of chronic, low-grade inflammation from an overactive immune system can be catastrophic. Going by the book, doctors hand out prescriptions that block the symptoms. But this masks the problem and often makes it worse. At best, it completely ignores the underlying disease.

If you take an NSAID to block your headache pain, the inflammation will simply crop up somewhere else. Since NSAIDs also disrupt the balance of bacteria in your gut, maybe the inflammation will manifest itself in gas or irritable bowel. Maybe your allergies will get worse. You may think there's just more pollen in the air, but if you weren't in a state of inflammation – taking pills that make it worse – the higher pollen level might not have affected you at all.

The trouble is that most doctors aren't thinking like medical detectives. They don't know to look at the whole body for signs of inflammation on the move, showing up in one symptom after another. They don't realize that, under the wrong circumstances, a single infection can flare into an autoimmune disorder like a brush fire out of control.

They don't realize that the body can develop a state of constant inflammation that can destroy your resilience, make your life miserable on a daily basis, and ultimately set you up for one of the new autoimmune diseases.

CHAPTER 6

—

ENVIRONMENTAL TOXINS

- *The top three toxins are molds, heavy metals, and glyphosates.*
- *Americans can no longer assume the water is safe to drink.*
- *The air in our homes, offices, and cars is often worse than the smoggiest cities.*

New research shows that when a pregnant mother is exposed to pollution, it can not only damage the immune system of her unborn child, but that damage will also be passed on to her children's children for generations.[137]

We're so accustomed to smoggy cities and toxin-spewing factories that we act as if it doesn't matter. But pollution is a serious thing. It poses a direct threat to the health of our children and ourselves. It is another trigger for autoimmunity.

We live in a toxic world, literally inhaling and consuming a soup of chemicals that do serious harm to our immune systems, both innate and acquired. Most of them directly damage our brains. When they pass through our intestines, they promote leaky gut, which sets us up for autoimmunity.[138] You may not get sick immediately, but if sufficient quantities are absorbed, inhaled, or ingested, you may fall prey to subtle changes in your health that you may not notice for years.[139]

The U.S. Department of Health and Human Services, Hazardous Substances Data Bank, lists specific products by brand name.[140] This short list is not at all comprehensive.

- **All canned food** (Bisphenol A) increases risk of obesity, heart disease and cancer.
- **Peanut butter** (Aflatoxin) produces Aspergillus fungus, causing liver disease and cancer.
- **Water-based cosmetics, deodorants** (Imidazolidine urea) emit formaldehyde.
- **Any soft plastics, insecticides, detergents** (Phthalates) disrupt hormones.
- **Antibacterial soap** causes thyroid disruption, hormonal imbalance, antibiotic resistance.
- **Nonstick cookware** (Perfluoroalkyl acid) causes ADHD, high cholesterol, infertility.
- **Dry cleaning** (Perchloroethylene) is a carcinogen and damages the nervous system.[141]

Identifying and ridding yourself of these poisons is essential for your total recovery. In my practice, very sick people come to me with diagnoses that are not responding to treatment. They are often suffering from toxic overload that no one imagined possible.

Everyone knows that we live in a toxic world, where our oceans, farms, food supply, the products we use, and the containers we store them in are often contaminated with mold, heavy metals, pesticides, mycotoxins, organic pollutants microplastics, and air pollution. Most of us avoid our own tap water out of a justified fear it may contain pesticides, lead, or dangerous bacteria.

We are surrounded by the toxins that fill our homes and offices – from cleaning fluids, toxic paints, carpets, and furniture. At room temperature, these products vaporize and become gas, or VOCs (volatile organic compounds). In the worst cases, they can burn our eyes, congest our noses, cause headaches, and make us wheeze: the body's way of telling us we are being poisoned.

AIR POLLUTION

Today, the air in our homes, offices, and automobiles is oftentimes worse than the most polluted cities.[142] The air quality in most buildings is less than ideal. Beyond the known pollution from smog, it can contain VOCs, gases emitted from furniture, carpeting, and building materials.

In 1970, the U.S. Congress formed the Environmental Protection Agency (EPA) and passed the Clean Air Act to regulate compounds that could endanger our health. In 1973, the EPA began a phased reduction of lead in gasoline after the Surgeon General found that exposure to lead could result in "chronic degenerative diseases." Anemia, behavioral disorders, low IQ, learning disabilities, and nerve damage afflicted children with toxic lead exposure. Adults suffered from hypertension and cardiovascular disease.[143]

The American Lung Association reports that one in four Americans (141 million people) live with air quality contamination from ozone and particle pollution that is unhealthful enough to put their health and lives at risk.[144]

Mercury is carried by the air of the marine fog off the beaches of California. Researchers at UC Santa Cruz found that the neurotoxin is carried by the fog, deposited on the land, and makes its way up the food chain. The mercury levels in the local puma population were three times higher than normal.[145]

Diesel exhaust in hair has definitively been shown to provoke neuroinflammation and increase levels of an abnormal protein called *amyloid-beta* that impairs brain function.[146]

Cleaner fuel would be helpful. By 1996, leaded fuel was banned completely for all vehicles on the road.[147] Two years later, the EPA found MTBE (methyl tertiary-butyl ether), which had also been used in gasoline, was contaminating the drinking water and impacting air quality. (To date, only 17 states have banned or limited its use.)[148] Both California and Denmark plan to phase it out.[149]

Unfortunately, in response to the reduction in lead, gasoline producers substituted BTEX (benzene, toluene, ethylbenzene, xylene) complex, which is also highly toxic and linked to developmental disorders, cancers, and neurodegenerative disorders, as well as cardio-pulmonary impairment. [150]

The disappearance of sparrows may be caused by the fumes from these toxins. Like canaries in the coal mines, the sparrows' demise coincides with the dramatic increase in MTBE and benzene. These birds, which lived alongside humans for more than 10,000 years, have declined by 70 percent since 1995[151] – in urban centers, *but not in small towns.*[152] As Dr. Denis Summers-Smith, the world authority on sparrows, wonders, "While the removal of lead from petrol was unquestionably right, could it be that it was at the cost of introducing other undesirable materials to the environment?"[153]

While many people assume that air filters in the cabins of their cars will protect them from pollution, that is not always the case. When they are changed regularly, standard filters do block large particles (pollen and dust) but are not designed to filter car emissions.

A study in *Environmental Health* found that factory-installed cabin air filters remove 46 percent of particulates, leaving nitrogen dioxide (NO_2) and hydrocarbon pollutants in the air. Buying a filter with activated carbon can reduce NO_2 and hydrocarbons by 75 percent and 50 percent, respectively.[154]

Setting the air conditioner to "recirculate" can reduce particulate pollutants in the car by 90 percent. But within 15 minutes, one or two people can exhale carbon dioxide in concentrations of 2,500 to 4,000 parts per million – enough to trigger drowsiness, headaches, poor decision-making, and even mild nausea (aka "car sickness"). So, it's important to turn the recirculating function off for a few minutes at regular intervals.[155]

WATER POLLUTION

Virtually all the drinking water in the United States comes from fresh surface waters and ground water aquifers. Surface waters and aquifers can be contaminated by various chemicals, microbes, and radionuclides. Disinfection of drinking water has dramatically reduced the prevalence of waterborne diseases (such as typhoid, cholera, hepatitis gastrointestinal illnesses, and chronic diseases such as cancer).[156]

After the shocking lead contamination in Flint, Michigan, *National Geographic* determined that it was not an isolated case. Americans can no longer assume the water is safe to drink. The EPA regulates 90 contaminants – but 100 more are unregulated.[157] In fact, 25 percent of our drinking water does not meet safety standards. The potential health impact is dire: potential "neurological problems and developmental disabilities in children (lead), interference with hormones (perchlorates), and increased risk of cancers of the skin, bladder, and kidney (arsenic)."[158]

As these risks grow, the appeal of bottled water grows stronger, particularly when the images on the ads and labels feature clear, sparkling mountain streams. But when the EPA studied ten major brands of bottled water in 2008, it found 38 pollutants from byproducts of the disinfection process to industrial chemicals to rampant bacteria and plastic particles. As things stand now, the best solution for lowering contamination appears to be well-filtered tap water.[159]

Both our salt water and fresh water supplies are at risk from mercury and microplastics. For years we have been aware of the presence of mercury in the oceans, but microplastics are now becoming an even more serious problem.

Since the 1950s, we have produced over eight billion tons of plastic, and we've recycled less than ten percent. Eventually, it ends up in the rivers, oceans, and air. Between eating, drinking, and breathing, we ingest 74,000 microplastic particles each year (about five grams a week, the size of a credit card).[160]

The effects of microplastics on our health are poorly understood, but we do know that in animals, microplastics can cross the blood-brain barrier. Most of them contain polychlorinated biphenyls (PCBs), which have been linked to cancer and immune system impairment. In animals, these particles reach the organs and deposit themselves in the gastrointestinal tract.[161]

TOP THREE TOXINS

If this summary seems overwhelming, imagine the volumes of books it would take to enumerate each and every poison we are commonly exposed to in our modern lives. It would be mind-boggling to say the least, so I'd like to narrow it down. In this chapter, we will mercifully focus only on the top three toxins I encounter in my practice:

1. Mold
2. Heavy metals
3. Glyphosate

1. MOLD

Mold contamination is the most common type of building-acquired infection. Inhaling mold spores can result in difficulty breathing. "If left untreated, mold contamination can spread through the bloodstream to other organs, resulting in death."[162]

Because mold represses the immune system, it interferes with healing, preventing the body from recovering from other problems and triggering autoimmune issues. It is estimated that 15 to 20 percent of respiratory conditions, such as allergic rhinitis, bronchitis, and asthma can be attributed to indoor mold.[163]

Mold is a nontechnical term for fungi that grows in places with water, food, and the proper temperature. The most common types of indoor mold are aspergillus, penicillin, cladosporium, alternaria, and stachybotrys chartarum (black mold). One type of stachybotrys chartarum is so toxic it is used as a chemical weapon.

Cellulose, which is an ideal food for mold, is found abundantly in the wallboards of our homes. Moisture can seep in due to rain leaks, groundwater leaks, or plumbing leaks. There may be stagnant water due to appliances, such as dishwashers, condensation coils, or the drip pans of HVAC systems.

Mold toxins are not only neurotoxins, which attack your brain, but they are also immunotoxins, which impair the ability of your body to fight other infections. Early evidence shows that mold toxins can cause your immune system to attack your own brain through the production of antibodies that attack – not other infections, as they should – but the nervous system tissue itself!

Exposure to toxic molds can cause a host of symptoms and diseases that most physicians never connect to mold, such as neurological diseases, autoimmune diseases, and cancers. They can even make you more susceptible to Multiple Chemical Sensitivity Disorder, in which exposure to even small amounts of different chemicals makes you sick.[164]

Molds naturally produce toxins, called mycotoxins, to protect themselves from other organisms in the environment. We are exposed to mycotoxins through the food we eat and the air we breathe. Like everything, our susceptibility to mycotoxins is determined by genetics, underlying health, and, of course, the amount and duration of exposure.

The extent of sensitivity to mycotoxins can vary quite dramatically from person to person. This is because of your genes. If you do not have the genes that produce the enzymes to breakdown mold toxins, you will get sick. I have treated a number of couples where one spouse was deathly ill from the mycotoxins in their house and the other had no problems whatsoever. In several cases, the one spouse was so sick trying to live in the house, that despite multiple attempts at treatment of the individual and remediation of the home, the couple was forced to move. Out of the moldy environment and with treatment, everyone was again healthy.

It is unfortunate, but sometimes a house is so contaminated with mold that the problem cannot be completely resolved. Many of the homes lost in New Orleans and Houston fell into this category.

If you suspect you may have been exposed to mold, these symptoms may provide clues:
- Chronic headaches
- Chronic fatigue
- Difficulty with memory
- Poor concentration or brain fog
- ADHD
- Depression
- Chronic joint or muscle pain
- Inability to regulate body temperature
- Inability to lose weight
- Asthma
- Allergies
- Frequent sinus or respiratory infections
- Abdominal pain
- Bloating

- Irregular stools
- Unusual nerve sensations, such as tingling or numbness
- Rashes or skin irritation
- Panic attacks
- Tremors
- Seizure-like symptoms
- Sensitivities to multiple chemicals, such as cleaning fluids or perfumes

The good news is that most people can rapidly clear mold toxins from their body. If they are removed from a mold-infested environment, they recover within a few days. Unfortunately, about 20 percent of people, for genetic reasons not yet completely understood, do not naturally clear the toxins from their bodies.

If there has been water damage to your home that has not been properly remediated, it is quite likely that you have a mold problem. Look for evidence of water damage to the ceiling, water marks on the walls, signs of black mold, and discolored heating or air vents. Notice whether your symptoms worsen on rainy or humid days. Keep in mind that if you have a central air heating and cooling system, any mold problem has most likely spread throughout the house.

Mold Testing

Wet drywall and wood are ideal environments for mold to grow. The toxic byproducts they release, called mycotoxins, can be responsible for serious health issues.

It is a significant problem throughout the United States. The average prevalence of mold in homes is at 45 percent.[165] It has also been a plague to college campuses as prestigious as Harvard and Georgetown. After the eradication of mold in Dunster House on the campus at Harvard in 2019, Zachary

M. Gingo, Associate Dean for Physical Resources and Planning for the Faculty of Arts and Sciences, pointed out, "It is important to know that mold and mildew are present in virtually all buildings."[166]

Unfortunately, many of these buildings are warehouses that store (and contaminate) the food we eat. Mycotoxins are commonly found in grains, coffee, cacao, peanuts, dried fruit, and spices. And, of course, the animals we eat are often fed that grain and pass it along to us in our meat, milk, and eggs. Eating a diet heavy in grains can increase overall burden of mycotoxins.[167]

Home testing kits are readily available, although you may need to hire an indoor air quality specialist who can evaluate your home more thoroughly. Testing and treatment are pretty straightforward. In most states, you can order mold toxin testing kits yourself, and many times you can eliminate the problem with simple and safe treatments that do not require you to see your physician. In the chapter on "Do it yourself," I have provided you with the tests and treatment protocols that may help.

2. HEAVY METALS

Have you ever noticed that multivitamins contain heavy metals? Many heavy metals are essential mineral elements that we need to maintain our bodily functions. Cobalt (Co), copper (Cu), chromium (Cr), iron (Fe), magnesium (Mg), manganese (Mn), molybdenum (Mo), nickel (Ni), selenium (Se), and zinc (Zn) all play important roles in reducing oxidation in our systems. We need them to live.[168]

That's why almost all of the cereals, breads, and crackers that we eat are fortified with iron. Without enough of these minerals, a host of diseases, such as red blood cell deficiency (anemia), can occur. Taking supplements containing heavy metals can help treat or prevent numerous diseases.[169] At the same time, toxic exposure to heavy metals can gradually suppress our immune systems and end in death. We are typically exposed to these toxic heavy metals though ingestion, inhalation, or skin contact.

Rather than expelling these toxins immediately, our bodies take the more cautious route of storing heavy metals, then excreting them slowly in order to minimize the potential for organ damage. But long-term storing or exposure of heavy metals can cause health problems, even if they are less dramatic than an acute reaction, such as that of a child accidentally swallowing mercury and immediately being rushed to the emergency room.[170] Lead, arsenic, chromium, and mercury are extremely toxic, even in small quantities.

As elements, heavy metals are at least five times denser than water. The degree of toxicity is related to the degree of elemental density. Due to their high degree of density and toxicity, mercury, lead, cadmium, chromium, titanium, and arsenic in our environment present significant health problems.[171]

Mercury Toxicity

Mercury is found naturally in air, soil, and water.[172] Over the past 20 years, mercury levels in the northern Pacific Ocean have risen 30 percent. It is predicted that they will rise 50 percent more by 2050, according to a study by researchers at the U.S. Geological Survey and Harvard University.[173]

Our exposure is rising along with it. When we eat seafood containing methylmercury, more than 95 percent of it passes into our bloodstreams, where it is absorbed, moving through the body, penetrating cells in every tissue and organ we have.[174]

Higher fish ingestion correlates with higher mercury levels, but not every fish is as hazardous as others. Choosing fish carefully can make a dramatic difference – six ounces of salmon (4 mcg mercury) vs. canned albacore tuna (60 mcg mercury) vs. swordfish (170 mcg mercury).[175]

The nutritional benefits of fish outweigh the risks of mercury exposure, but the Food and Drug Administration recommends that pregnant or breastfeeding women keep the following recommendations in mind:

- Eat 2–3 servings (227–340 grams) of a variety of fish every week.
- Choose lower-mercury fish, such as salmon, shrimp, cod, and sardines.
- Avoid higher-mercury fish, such as tilefish, shark, swordfish, and king mackerel.
- Look out for fish advisories for particular streams or lakes that source fish.[176]

Lead Toxicity

Lead can find its way into drinking water through lead pipes, faucets, or fixtures in the home or the water main, which is the most significant source of lead in water. To limit your exposure:

- Use only cold water from the tap (boiling does not remove the lead).
- Clean your faucet's screen (aerator) on a regular basis.
- Add a water filter certified to remove lead. Replace the filter on time.
- Run the tap before you drink, shower, or do laundry to flush the pipes.
- Contact your water services to learn more about local sources of lead.

3. GLYPHOSATE

Glyphosate is the most widely used herbicide in the United States. As many as 100 million pounds a year is sprayed on agriculture and suburban lawns. Monsanto's popular weed-killing product, Roundup, contains glyphosate, but studies show it is far more toxic to human cells than that ingredient alone.[177]

Roundup contains an inert ingredient that can literally suffocate human cells. This fact has sparked an intense debate about substances that are called "inerts," but are often much more harmful than anticipated. Solvents, preservatives, surfactants, and other substances are added to pesticides as a matter of course, but are now being seen as health hazards in themselves.[178]

Nearly 4,000 inert ingredients are approved for use by the EPA. Because they have been assumed to be "inert," they have been less scrutinized for safety than active ingredients. Many are not even disclosed to the EPA because they are protected as trade secrets. Yet a new study shows that Roundup's inerts amplify glyphosate's toxic effect on human cells, even when tested at much lower concentrations than are commonly used.[179]

Monsanto scientists have attempted to argue that the study tested levels that were much higher than real-world exposure; the doses tested actually ranged from the standard agricultural dose to concentrations that were 100,000 times more diluted than the products sold in stores. At every level, despite the concentration of Roundup, cell damage occurred. Glyphosate and the inerts in this product literally limited the capacity of the cells to breathe, stressed them out, and drove them toward suicide.[180] Clearly, weeds aren't the only thing this popular product kills.

Monsanto introduced Roundup in 1974. Yet this is the first time the U.S. National Toxicology Program (NTP) has tested weed killing formulas that contain glyphosate along with other chemicals. Glyphosate was previously tested in isolation, but government scientists approved the sale of glyphosate amplified by other chemicals to consumers and farmers without testing it more than 40 years ago.[181]

Today geneticists, in conjunction with farmers, worldwide have ensured that more than 80 percent of genetically modified (GM) crops are resistant to Roundup. The weed killer is meant to kill all plant life except the GM crops. Instead, weeds have become resistant to glyphosate, resulting in super weeds that are exceptionally hard to kill. Farmers have responded by spraying more and more glyphosate on their GM crops. When that does not work, they resort to the notoriously toxic herbicides that were abandoned a generation ago because of their noxious effects, such as 2,4-Dichlorophenoxyacetic acid, one of the ingredients in the Vietnam War's defoliant Agent Orange.[182]

With so little concern for the human beings being poisoned along with the weeds, it is inevitable that the effects on our health are coming to light. It is now suspected that glyphosate triggers autoimmunity diseases such as celiac when it is sprayed on wheat, one of the most common ingredients in all processed foods in America.[183]

Glyphosate damages the microvilli in the gut, reducing their ability to absorb vitamins and minerals. Because it is not recognized by the body and cannot be broken down, it is even more likely to provoke an immunological response. Autism, autoimmune diseases, cancer, Parkinson's, Alzheimer's, inflammatory bowel diseases (Crohn's and ulcerative colitis), cardiovascular, depression, and infertility have all been linked to glyphosate.[184]

Because it chelates essential minerals, the gut microbes do not have access to them. This results in a chronic state of inflammation, which as we know, is behind all chronic illness.

Any time we eat processed food, we are eating glyphosate. It cannot be washed off. It is infused into every cell of the plant. The only way to keep your diet free of glyphosate is to:

- Avoid conventionally grown and processed foods
- Eat meat that was not fed GMO grains, since glyphosate accumulates in animal tissues
- Eat organic butter and dairy for the same reason
- Eat an organic diet
- Take a multi-mineral supplement that includes trace minerals
- Support glutathione production with N-acetylcysteine, glycine and glutamine
- Support liver detoxification by avoiding alcohol
- Support liver health by taking silymarin and lipoid acid[185]

The Think Dirty app can help you identify which products to avoid before you buy them. You can scan the products, learn their ingredients, then choose to shop for clean options.
https://www.thinkdirtyapp.com/

CHAPTER 7

—

EMOTIONAL TRAUMA

- *Trauma can have a significant negative impact on health for decades.*
- *Not all stress is traumatic. It may be positive, tolerable, or toxic.*
- *Childhood trauma is linked to the leading causes of death among adults.*

Whether it happened this afternoon or many years ago, emotional trauma can leave you in a state of prolonged stress that undermines your immune system and makes your odds of getting autoimmunity much higher.

The profound, complex, and fascinating relationship between our emotional health and our immunological health goes both ways. Our mood affects the first responders of the innate immune system and the defense team of the acquired immune system.

Trauma can have long-lasting effects on our physical, social, and emotional health.[186] For years, studies have shown that emotional trauma is a potential set-up for the development of life-threatening infections[187] and autoimmune disorders.[188] It can even increase the risk of neurodegenerative disorders, such as multiple sclerosis, Parkinson's, and Alzheimer's.[189]

Our immune systems are extremely sensitive to stress. When we experience any kind of trauma, they are immediately impacted.

The American Psychological Association defines trauma as "an emotional response to a terrible event like an accident, rape, or natural disaster."[190] Trauma specialist Dr. Peter Levine makes an important distinction between the event itself and the emotional reaction that follows. In his view, trauma can be "...*any* overwhelming and distressing experience." Since people's reactions to the same event are so varied, the experience and the symptoms afterward are the only way to distinguish between what was traumatic and what was not.[191]

Often there is no visible sign of injury when an emotional trauma occurs. The emotional toll may not show up until years later. Huge physical events like earthquakes, car accidents, wildfires, hurricanes, and tsunamis can cause emotional trauma just as much as personal tragedy, loss, heartbreak, abuse, and neglect.

Events that traumatize large sections of the population – such as the coronavirus, terrorist attacks, school shootings, assassinations, or natural disasters – are often followed by *epidemics* of survivor's guilt and post-traumatic stress disorder.

A volcanic eruption can occur so suddenly, with such overwhelming force, that a person's first reaction is often shock, then numbness or denial. All three of these reactions serve to force reality away, to keep the thought of it at a safe distance as much as possible. Once the immediate crisis is over and the status quo has been restored or they have found a place of relative safety, they can relax that defense. When they do, they may be flooded with the frightened, horrified emotions their mind has been saving for later. High levels of guilt, anxiety, or depression may come over them.

Their bodies are swamped with the stress hormone cortisol, which is automatically released in trauma. It triggers what is commonly known as the fight-or-flight response. In a volcanic eruption, flight is almost certainly the right response, but if the trauma is severe, it can permanently damage the ability of the immune system to control the release of cortisol. The inflammation that results can lead to any number of diseases from heart disease to diabetes to autoimmune disorders.[192]

It's normal to experience traumatic stress following a disturbing event, whether it's the coronavirus pandemic, a traffic accident, plane crash, violent crime, terrorist attack, or a natural disaster like an earthquake, hurricane, or flood. You may feel intense shock, confusion, and fear, or feel numb or overwhelmed by a host of conflicting emotions, sometimes all at once. And these emotions aren't limited to the people who experienced the event. Round-the-clock news and social media coverage means that we're all bombarded with horrific images of tragedy, suffering, and loss almost the instant they occur anywhere in the world. Repeated exposure can overwhelm your nervous system and create traumatic stress just as if you experienced the event first-hand.

Traumatic stress can shatter your sense of security, leaving you feeling helpless and vulnerable in a dangerous world – especially if the traumatic event was manmade, such as a shooting or act of terrorism. You may feel physically and emotionally drained, overcome with grief, or find it difficult to focus, sleep, or control your temper. These are all normal responses to abnormal events.

Often, the unsettling thoughts and feelings of traumatic stress – as well as any unpleasant physical symptoms – start to fade as life gradually returns to normal over the days or weeks following a catastrophic event or crisis. But there's also a lot you can do to assist in your recovery and better come to terms with the trauma you've experienced. Whether you lived through the event itself, witnessed it, were an emergency responder or medical worker, or experienced traumatic stress in the aftermath, there are plenty of ways to calm your nervous system and regain your emotional balance.[193]

The brain is also impacted by trauma. Lasting changes can take place in the amygdala, the hippocampus, and the prefrontal cortex that can impair brain functioning. Until the mind has had a chance to work through the trauma and process the emotions, the excessive cortisol release can actually rewire the circuits of the brain in ways that change reactions and perceptions.

Anyone who has experienced a severe injury, illness, natural disaster, crime, surgical procedure, community violence, sexual abuse, physical abuse, domestic violence, neglect, deprivation, traumatic grief, accident, attack, school violence, fire, flood, or loss of any kind has been traumatized.[194] The crucial variable is: how did they react?

The impact on the brain, the emotions, and the body itself is profoundly different, depending on who the person is, what their age is, and which of the three types of trauma occurred:

- **Acute trauma** happens once (such as a train wreck or an attack).
- **Chronic trauma** happens repeatedly over hours, days, or years (such as domestic violence or emotional abuse).
- **Complex trauma** happens relentlessly in varied, invasive, traumatic events (such as a prisoner of war camp or a home with mentally ill parents).[195]

Acute trauma triggers an intense physiological response. All the chemicals provoked by the event work to sear into the brain a link between the trauma and the pain or fear experienced along with it. For most people, those feelings and associations gradually dissipate with the help of supportive loved ones and friends. Less than ten percent of people are unable to shake it off without additional help. If the traumatic associations interfere with their ability to function for more than a month, it qualifies as post-traumatic stress disorder.[196]

PTSD has a host of effects on the body's physiology.[197] Plagued by fearful memories of the event, PTSD sufferers begin to avoid anything that might trigger those memories: a location, an activity, a song, a scent. The body knows it was unable to fully return to health after the event(s), so it becomes hyper-vigilant to protect itself. As a result, it leaves the victim in a heightened state of arousal, always on the lookout for a similar event.[198] Understandably, many people with PTSD gradually develop severe depression, even suicidal thoughts, and problems with addictions.

In 2018, the *Journal of the American Medical Association* (JAMA) published a 30-year study of over 100,000 patients, showing that those with stress-related disorders had a significantly greater risk of contracting an autoimmune disease than their siblings without these disorders. Although their experience is different from that of most of the population in the United States, a recent study of Vietnam War veterans confirms that those who had PTSD were more likely to develop autoimmune diseases. The same is true of people with more common stress-related disorders.[199]

Most people who experience life stressors, such as violence, life-threatening events, or the loss of a loved one, gradually recover, but many develop severe emotional problems, such as post-traumatic stress disorder (PTSD), acute stress disorder (ASD), or adjustment disorder (AD). While each of those reactions has a strong emotional component, there are also clearly discernible physical changes. The hypothalamic-pituitary-adrenal axis and the autonomic nervous system may be disrupted, leading to impairment of the immune system. The body's inflammatory reflex can become over-reactive. Low cortisol levels are common and can result in an increase in inflammatory cytokines, accelerated aging of immune cells, and a hyperactive immune system. Lifestyle changes such as substance abuse or sleep disruption are also common and can lead to autoimmune disease.[200]

CHILDHOOD TRAUMA

Coping with adversity is vital for the development of any healthy child. When stress occurs in a supportive environment of primary relationships with adults, it is mollified and contained in ways that promote the development of healthy stress response systems.

When there are no support systems available, the child is genetically or temperamentally vulnerable, or the stress is too extreme and long-lasting, recovery from the emotional trauma is harder. It can result instead in lifelong damage to the brain, chronic inflammation, and overall system impairment. [201]

The Center for the Developing Child at Harvard University identifies three responses to stress: positive, tolerable, and toxic.

- **Positive:** Essential to healthy development. Stress that causes brief increases in heart rate and mild hormonal elevations (falling in love, meeting a new caregiver).
- **Tolerable:** Damaging. Severe stress that fires off major alerts in the body (the loss of a loved one, a near-death experience). Although it is extreme, it is acute (a one-time event). If it is buffered by loving, supportive relationships, the brain and body recover well.
- **Toxic.** Long-Lasting. More extreme stress caused by prolonged adversity (caregiver abuse, exposure to violence, accumulated burdens of family economic hardship). This level of trauma can disrupt brain and organ

development, resulting in an increased risk for injuries, autoimmune diseases, and early death later in life.[202]

Adults and children can experience any of these responses to stress, but children younger than six years old are far more vulnerable to trauma because their brains are in a formative stage. If a child is exposed to chronic trauma or complex trauma, the brain develops with its neurological patterns in a permanently heightened state. Survival is prioritized to new levels. Emotional, behavioral, and cognitive changes take place to increase its ability to cope with extreme stress, without support, on an ongoing basis. Other functions are minimized or even sacrificed to devote as many resources to survival as possible. As the traumatic experiences continue, it not only shapes the child's behavior but also the child's mental and emotional development, as well as their long-term physical health.[203]

Adults who grew up with toxic stress can have difficulty forming healthy relationships, maintaining employment, ensuring stable finances, and keeping their emotional equilibrium. Not only can these symptoms be passed on to their own children, but they also may well have begun their own lives at a disadvantage through inherited trauma.[204]

According to the Centers for Disease Control and Prevention (CDC), Adverse Childhood Experiences (ACEs) are common. In a survey of adults in 25 states, 61 percent reported at least one ACE. Almost one in six reported four or more ACEs.[205] In the United States, nearly 1,770 children died of abuse and neglect in 2018. The rate is five times higher in families with low socio-economic status.[206]

As we begin to correlate ACEs with health conditions, it becomes clear that we could prevent as many as 1.9 million cases of heart disease and 21 million cases of depression by preventing ACEs.[207]

In fact, ACEs impact all these areas: physical injury from all causes, mental health, ill-health in pregnancy, infectious disease, chronic disease, risk-taking behavior, and loss of opportunities in work and life.[208]

The ACE STUDY

In 1998, a major study of over 13,000 adults found that childhood abuse and family dysfunction was linked to many of the leading causes of death in adults.[209]

The ACEs they focused on fell into seven categories: psychological, physical, or sexual abuse, witnessing violence against their mother, and having members of the household who were substance abusers, mentally ill, suicidal, or imprisoned.

Adults who had been exposed to many of these ACEs in childhood were strongly at risk for bone fractures, heart disease, chronic lung disease, cancer, and liver disease.

The risk did not result from what we have called Acute Trauma, but a toxic response to Complex Trauma. The study showed an unequivocally strong relationship between "the breadth of exposure" to abuse or family dysfunction in childhood and multiple risks for the leading causes of death in adults.[210] A strong experience of trauma may reduce life expectancy by as much as 20 years.[211]

ADVERSE CHILDHOOD EXPERIENCE TEST

Knowing your ACE score can help you protect yourself. The Stop Abuse Campaign at stopabusecampaign.org offers this ACE test called: What is Your ACE Score?

https://stopabusecampaign.org/faq-the-ace-study/what-is-your-ace-score/

The ACEs on this test fall into in three categories; abuse, neglect, and family dysfunction. Afterward, the site describes your health risks and offers strategies for prevention of ACEs. As ACEs increase, so does bad health, either now or later. As the Stop Abuse Campaign so aptly says: childhood trauma has adult consequences.[212]

More than one in ten people score four or more on this ten-question ACE Test. A score of four means four-fold increase in the likelihood of becoming a substance abuser. The risk of chronic depression or serious work issues is tripled. Serious financial problems, heart disease, or stroke are twice as likely to occur. A score of five to ten makes the risk of suicide nine times greater.[213]

FALSE MEMORIES

After decades of debate about whether a memory of a trauma or series of traumas can be forgotten for years, then suddenly remembered, and whether a "memory" can be suggested, then remembered as true, The American Psychological Association has this to say.

> Both phenomena occur. Most leaders in the field agree that recovered memory is an extremely rare event, but it is possible. It is also possible to construct emotionally powerful memories of events that never occurred. The mechanisms involved in memory are not yet well understood. And without corroborating evidence, we have no way to distinguish a true memory from a false one.[214]

Unfortunately, the possibility of repressed vs. suggested memories have been sensationalized by the media. The stories we are most familiar with portray the least likely possibility of all: total amnesia of a childhood trauma that is suddenly remembered. Instead, most victims of childhood trauma have always remembered part or all of what happened, and it is sometimes possible to retrieve more details about those partial memories.[215]

But there is, again, very little need or reason to believe that those details are strictly accurate. All of our memories are modified by outside factors whether we're aware of it or not. As strange as it seems, it is the nature of memory to change and adjust to our ongoing experience of life.

Ultimately, the details are no more important to emotional recovery than the details of a natural disaster or car accident are important to recovery. The trauma lies in the emotional response, not the event itself. Healing and recovery come from treating the emotional trauma so you can be free of the toxic experiences in the past and live a full, healthy life.

Are old beliefs getting in the way of your healing?

As I mentioned in *Total Recovery*, I once had the privilege of attending a lecture by Dr. Elizabeth Kubler Ross shortly after medical school. This lecture had such a profound and lasting impression on me that it has shaped my practice of medicine to this day.

Dr. Elizabeth Kubler Ross, a world-renowned psychiatrist, was the author of numerous papers and books, the most famous of which is *On Death and Dying*. In this book, Dr. Kubler Ross outlined the five stages of death in which we move from denial to acceptance of our fate.

In the lecture, Dr. Kubler Ross discussed her work with a young man who was dying of cancer. He had undergone several treatments with chemotherapy that were unsuccessful, and the cancer specialist had referred the young man to Dr. Kubler Ross to help him process and accept his fate. She asked the gentleman to draw a picture, which she shared with us, of his experience with the chemotherapy.

The illustration depicted the cancer cells as meek, mild creatures that were being viciously attacked by the chemotherapy medications. Underneath the picture he had written, "Thou shall not kill." He was a Quaker, and his interpretation of his belief was such that even if something was killing him, it would be against God's will for him to kill.

Dr. Kubler Ross spent some time examining this belief with him, and after several sessions he drew another picture that now depicted the chemotherapy medications as gentle, monk-like creatures lifting the cancer cells and escorting the cancer out of his body.

She reported that he returned for another round of chemotherapy and this time the medications worked and his cancer went into remission.

There is no separation of mind and body. If we are to heal from devastating chronic illness, we must free up all our internal healing resources and use all the necessary medical resources to recover. This young man would have died too soon had it not been for the wisdom and skill of Dr. Kubler Ross and his oncologist.

Chronic illness can be a type of death. We are taken off our life's path and forced into the role of illness. You may have lost the ability to continue schooling or work. Your ability to interact with friends and family is impaired, and in some cases, lost. There are days you cannot get out of bed and days filled with pain and disability.

There is a path forward for you. Our understanding of why you are suffering with chronic Lyme disease, chronic pain, chronic fatigue, chronic depression and anxiety, POTS, PANS, and PANDAS has changed, and hope is now a real thing.

PART III

HORROR STORIES WITH HAPPY ENDINGS

The root of all health is in the brain. The trunk of it is in emotion. The branches and leaves are the body. The flower of health blooms when all parts work together.

~ Old Kurdish saying

* * *

These are the stories of four of my patients as we worked together to heal their bodies from the infections that triggered autoimmune disease in them with devastating consequences.

Each chapter will begin with the medical horror stories endured by Sarah, Emily, Nathan, and Janet. They are followed by my observations, evaluations, recommendations, and treatments.

Regaining their health has given each of them back their lives. As you read their stories, notice the stages they went through, the way we peeled back the layers together to eliminate every single element that was damaging their health, and then calmed their immune systems so they could function normally again.

Your story will inevitably be different. Everyone's is. But the powerful approach to restoring your health will be the same as it was for them: Eliminate the infection and everything setting it up, then restore the immune system.

CHAPTER 8

—

SARAH | STRANGE SYMPTOMS OF INFECTION

As told by her mother

When Sarah was nine, she was a delight. As her mother, I knew her to be a compassionate, loving, sensitive child. Then she came down with what looked like Bell's palsy (BP). We spent a little more than two years going to doctors, getting nowhere, until finally we learned that it was being caused by Lyme disease.

Sarah was put on two weeks of antibiotics. Her palsy resolved, but she complained of hearing strange noises, beeping sounds. Something wasn't right. The local infectious disease doctor poo-pooed her symptoms.

From November 2012 until January 2013, she got better for a while; then she got very sick again and ended up with an impacted colon, no feeling in her legs, seizures, transient episodes of blindness, deafness, and the inability to speak. She would lose consciousness 40–50 times a day. At times, she would collapse on the floor in total body paralysis.

In 2013, she was diagnosed with POTS and Lyme. We had never seen a tick or a red bull's eye patch on her skin. Bell's palsy was first indication that something was going on. She was given antibiotics, but she continued to lose weight. She was always cold. It was nearly impossible to keep her hands and feet warm. Soon I was having to dress her every day.

By the end of 2013, she was bed-bound, unable to go to school, read, or write. Sarah was a shell of herself. She reverted to nonverbal sounds, OCD behavior, age-regression, eating weird objects, scanning for knives, autistic behavior, violent behaviors to herself and others, and lack of recognition of me in particular. She was hallucinating and hypersensitive to light, sound, and touch. She howled that we were screaming when we were whispering. When she was verbal, she'd swear I wasn't her mother, but an impostor.

We rushed her to all the major hospitals, to Johns Hopkins, to private neurologists. Nothing worked fully. We understood that the doctors didn't have answers, but it was unforgivable that they were not even curious. We felt betrayed by a medical system that was making no attempt to help us.

Before long, things became more dangerous. At times we didn't feel safe with her in our home. Sarah would scan a room for sharp objects – toys, wood, anything – then start jabbing them at people's faces with a very strange look on her own face. Sometimes she would try to put a knife through her own forehead in a jabbing motion or engage in in rapid OCD motions, chopping things into little pieces over and over again. Obviously, we soon hid the knives, but she would just continue the assaults with pillows, books, or laptops. She'd be fine one day, then get aggressive with family members out of nowhere. Eventually, we had to put her in lock holds to keep her down. It was very disturbing.

I went on a mission to figure out what the hell was happening with my daughter. It always pointed back to BP and

Lyme, but doctors all said it was impossible that it could still be inflammation from Lyme because she had had three weeks of antibiotics and the Lyme was surely dead. My mother's intuition told me otherwise.

That's when I started my relentless research. After she finally went to sleep each night, I spent my time furiously Googling, trying to find answers. It was online that I came across a document called *Under Our Skin* that told the stories of patients with symptoms that seemed a lot like Sarah's.

GETTING HELP

By 2014, the last Lyme doctor we saw in D.C. said she had no doubt that Sarah's condition was the result of a tick-borne disease. In fact, Sarah was showing the all the symptoms of this doctor's sickest patients. She never had seen any patient with all the symptoms. We needed more advanced help. She sent us to her mentor, Dr. Charles Ray Jones.

The soonest appointment available at his office was three months away, but in January 2015, my husband took Sarah on the train in a wheelchair with a nurse accompanying them. By this time, Sarah was so weak that we wondered whether she could endure a five-hour train ride. We knew it would be arduous.

Once Dr. Jones had a chance to examine her, he immediately put us at ease. He confirmed the diagnosis that it was tick-borne. It was more complicated for Sarah because, as he explained, "The Lyme infection has induced autoimmune encephalopathy. It can be healed but it will take a long time."

After waiting another month for lab tests and results, the blood work showed that Sarah's immune system was still intact. This was good news, he said. It meant that there was hope that he could help her. It felt like a moment of sunlight streaming through an opening in a perpetually dark sky.

But as the months passed, Dr. Jones tried numerous protocols, gave her many rounds of supplements, engaged in consultations with other specialists, and ran a series of MRIs and other brain scans costing thousands of dollars. Nothing was ever conclusive.

At this point, we felt she was dying. Every system in her body was shutting down. We couldn't understand how someone could lose consciousness so many times a day and survive for long. She had spent the last ten months in misery with no joy, no school days, no peers, no friends. She couldn't even speak without intense attacks of pain. What kind of life was this?

Slowly taking shape like an unwelcomed figure emerging from the fog was the sobering realization that I'd rather she was dead than live like this.

BREAKTHROUGH

And then we had a breakthrough. We were sent to Dr. David Younger, a neurologist at New York University, for a full brain workup.

By this time, my delightful, engaging daughter had retreated into herself almost completely. She presented cognitively like a severely autistic child. When Dr. Younger saw her oppositional behavior, he said she needed to see Dr. Eric Hollander, a psychiatrist, who could provide medication to alleviate her psychological issues, so Dr. Younger could complete the numerous tests he needed to perform.

We saw Dr. Hollander within days. He put her on a medication commonly used for schizophrenia, Zyprexa, explaining carefully that he did not believe Sarah had a mental disease, but an underlying medical condition. The drug sedated her enough to make nine days of intensive testing possible.

They did blood work, sleep studies, stress EEGs, tilt tables, electromagnetic studies using electrical current to test nerve response, skin-core biopsies on the thighs and calves of both legs to be evaluated by the Mayo Clinic, and spinal puncture.

Ironically, one of the basic tests Dr. Younger used for brain inflammation and its connection to tick-borne was a SPECT study where you're injected with dye and 45 minutes later an image is taken. During that imaging Sarah convulsed on the table, so the film was blurry. But it ended up being a lucky break.

Since that test was clearly too long for Sarah to tolerate, he did a PET study instead. It required a ten-minute instead of a 45-minute scan time.

The PET scan showed inflammation on the left side of her brain.

"Ironically, if she hadn't had the seizure," Dr. Younger said, "we might not have had a clear diagnosis. Because the PET scan showed it and the longer scan would not have." The PET scan is more detailed and deeper, but it's much more expensive. The machine is much larger. Perhaps the level of radiation might be greater. Insurance companies don't like to pay for it, so it's not a doctor's first choice. But NYU was a phenomenal hospital with wonderful resources.

What showed up in blood was co-infection, Bartonella, Babesia, and Lyme in her spinal fluid. Other causes of brain inflammation, such as anti-NMDA encephalitis, were ruled out, but her skin biopsy showed less than one-fifth of one percent of distal nerve leg fibers than normal for someone her age. Studies of the nerve connections to her muscles (EMG) were abnormal. POTS on the tilt table test, and her heart rate and her BP were off.

The official diagnosis: *chronic inflammatory demyelinating polyneuropathy* (CIDP).

LUCK STARTS TO CHANGE

Our relief at having a convincing diagnosis was profound. Since the treatment would involve regular infusions, Dr. Younger inserted a PICC line, a catheter that is temporarily left in place. This meant that there were even more serious restrictions to what she could do, including cautious bathing or physical contact, to protect the PICC line.

We would need a local doctor in Baltimore to supervise its use. Every local doctor and pediatrician we had seen had ultimately walked away. Our own family pediatrician, a doctor from Johns Hopkins, vehemently disagreed with the treatment and refused to participate. We didn't know where to turn.

That's when it seemed our luck finally started to change. "How close are you to D.C.?" Dr. Younger asked, and he referred us to Dr. Gary Kaplan.

It ended up being a phenomenal gift for our family. I feel like it was after we met with Dr. Kaplan that things started turning around. In our complex situation, he stepped in to oversee the various medical practitioners and treatments, bringing them all into conversation with one another. As we had repeatedly discovered, getting specialists to talk to one another is nearly impossible. Dr. Kaplan took charge of that, picking up the phone for conference calls, making the decisions, and rallying the minds together. It was exactly the help we had been missing.

Sarah's treatment relied on coordinating the protocols of Dr. Younger, the neurologist, and Dr. Jones, the Lyme specialist. It wasn't long before their opinions clashed.

Dr. Younger treated the infection for two months, while Dr. Jones insisted that two months wasn't enough.

Both believed that Sarah needed immune modulating therapy IV-IG, a mix of immunoglobulin donor plasma from 1,000 donors that had been spun, then irradiated. Sarah had been sick for so long that her immune system had started to make antibodies against her own nerves. The goal of giving her IV-IG was to quiet her immune system to get it to stop making antibodies against her own nervous system.

It was Dr. Jones' opinion that during IV-IG monthly infusions, Lyme patients needed to continue antibiotics to cover any infections that had not been irradiated out of the plasma. There were risks to this course of action. The CDC advised against it. We didn't know what to do.

Dr. Kaplan mediated with the doctors. His own medical view was aligned with Dr. Younger's two-month treatment, but he pointed out that Dr. Johns had 40 years of clinical experience in this area. As long as we were willing to take the risk, he recommended that we follow Dr. Jones' advice. So, we continued with antibiotics for about ten months.

We have never regretted it. Sarah started to heal in dramatic, miraculous ways. There is no doubt in our minds that she needed IV antibiotics for Lyme. She started on April 14, 2018. April 21 was the last day she ever used the wheelchair.

Instead of shouldering the burden alone, we had the help we needed at last. Dr. Kaplan has been an incredible communicator. He is curious, calling and learning from the other doctors as we go. He has also looked at things like organic acid tests in the urine, mold, or other imbalances, and has prescribed supplements to handle those.

When he found Sarah had mast cell activation, he gave her supplements to help her immune system to stay calmer. She's tried many medications to help with the inflammation or to calm the hyper-vigilance of her brain, but unfortunately, all of them failed. She's always had hypersensitivity and diabolical responses.

He thinks about things like whether long-term antibiotics are going to cause other problems, especially in the intestines.

He's prescribed probiotics, made dietary recommendations, and monitored the health of her intestines – things we would not have even thought about.

Most importantly, he does not just look at her physical symptoms, but he talks to her and asks about social issues, encouraging her to get out more with her friends. His emotional support, as someone she can talk with about her feelings, has provided incredible peace for our family.

We are glad to have a team with a physician treating us and our daughter as whole people. It's not as easy to measure that contribution, but it's priceless and goes a long way in getting well, especially in an illness that isn't understood and which has no clear-cut protocol.

For years we were alone, trying to contend with doctors who didn't agree with each other. There is immeasurable value in the feeling that your doctor and even the nurses in his office taking the blood are watching closely, looking for clues, and thinking about the whole problem.

MOLD

One of the other concerns Dr. Kaplan raised was the possibility of mold toxicity. He explained that many of his patients with chronic Lyme also had problems with other environmental toxins such as mold. Mold toxins can impair the immune system, making fighting off the Lyme tougher, and the toxins can also have a direct effect, causing inflammation in the brain. He ran testing on Sarah, but also recommended that we have the house checked for mold contamination and referred us to a company that tests indoor air quality.

It seemed unlikely that we would have a mold problem. We were living in a two-million-dollar home that we believed had been built to the highest standards. Still, we followed his advice and had our home tested. To our amazement, they found black mold.

We had had some water leaks that we thought we'd fixed, but clearly not. When the mold testing came back, the person who had tested the house for mold toxins told us to get out of the house and not to take anything with us, since it could all be contaminated. "Leave with nothing – as if your house were on fire." We did.

That was the week Sarah walked again. We didn't know for sure if her improvement had been the result of the antibiotic infusions or getting away from the mold, but it was a moment we will never forget.

We rented an apartment, started again, and never looked back, writing off everything we owned in it. It may sound incredible, but when your child is as ill as she was, it doesn't matter.

The experience has made us hyper-vigilant about looking for mold. When Sarah's symptoms returned last spring, we saw a hairline crack in her wall. I had a contractor open the wall up to find out what was going on. Incredibly, the contractor found mold.

In Maryland, we'd had rains unprecedented in 150 years. There was a chimney running down through Sarah's room. Water was coming in behind her walls. At least this time we were able to catch it early enough that we didn't need to permanently abandon the house.

We did need to leave while the mold was removed. Initially, we tried a hotel, but Sarah didn't feel well there. So, we moved the whole family into a tent on our deck outside. (We couldn't pitch the tent on the grass because of ticks.) When we had had about all we could take of living in a tent, we went on vacation. It was kind of a crazy situation, but we made the best of it.

Water can infiltrate a house at any time. We had to do a complete de/reconstruction of one side of the house, then we moved back in around December. All of Sarah's belongings had to be cleaned. We replaced her mattress and the upholstered bedframe. Anything made of porous or made of fabric had to be discarded, since her reaction had been severe.

WITCH HUNT

In February 2016, we had another crisis. The PICC line that threads up Sarah's arm to her heart broke!

When I tried to flush the line as I'd been shown, she started bleeding. It was gushing out fast. When I couldn't stop it, I called the infusion nurse who helped me know what to do, then we rushed to the emergency room.

They took Sarah in right away to stop the bleeding, but then things took a turn for the worse. I slammed into a wall of disdain, judgment, and bias from the medical staff. Like my local pediatrician, they were completely opposed to IV antibiotic treatment of this kind and didn't hesitate to make that very clear. They started grilling me with questions that were increasingly hostile, as I tried to explain her treatments. Exchanging troubling glances, they wanted to know who had recommended such a protocol and what their credentials were. The whole thing was quickly turning into a witch hunt.

When I called Dr. Kaplan, he advised me to tell them to remove the wire, then reinsert a new wire, but hold the line. They refused to do it. Again, they said they didn't agree with the diagnosis or treatment, even though I told them her story and success. I was very emotional and frustrated, as was Sarah. We both knew she had regained so much.

Dr. Kaplan tried speaking to the doctors himself, but they didn't budge. Finally, he told me, "We're not going to win this fight. Just remove the line. Maybe this is a sign that we need to take a break." He assured me that if she needed more, he would make sure we had the line reinstalled.

We continued with the IV-IG, but that was the end of the PICC line antibiotics. In the end, she continued taking IV-IG for three-and-a-half years and long-term oral antibiotics until November 2018.

To our amazement and relief, Sarah held her own. She started back to school in 2019 and is doing well.

RETURN TO LIFE

So much about being this sick is traumatic. She is still benefiting from the care of a renowned psychiatrist in New Jersey to help her recover emotionally, avoid denial, and learn coping skills. I kept coming across his fascinating medical journal articles while I was Googling Sarah's condition. He addresses changes to the brain that occur in relation to memory, processing, hyper-stimulation, and non-restorative sleep.

While Sarah's sleep has improved enormously, thanks to the drug Trazadone, her processing and cognitive abilities are lingering challenges. So, it is with a real sense of accomplishment that she is able to do a full academic day now. For all the traumas she endured, she only lost one year of school when she was bed-bound.

Reading, walking, hearing, seeing, talking, emotional stability – it's all returned. We are slowly getting our daughter back.

One physician told me, "It's not going to be this terrible and get better right away. Try to string together more good days than bad. It will be up and down. But if you focus on that, you can start to see the progress." He was right.

When we went back to Dr. Younger for follow-up testing, he repeated the electric frequency test. Her results, which had shown extremely abnormal impaired leg function, were now completely normal. He said that her nerve regeneration was a benefit of youth. Had she been 50 years old, she might never have fully regained function based on the damage. We were very happy about her level of recovery.

Today, Sarah is back on the competitive cheerleading team, jumping in the air with her friends, and doing back flips. The joy of seeing her do a five-trick gymnastic move after all of this will never leave me. For longer than I care to remember, I lived with the fear that she would soon be dead or permanently in a wheelchair.

But now, in 2019, she has gotten her life back.

WHAT I KNOW NOW

People ask me what I know now that I wish I'd known when all of this began.

It sounds obvious, but it's not: Do not underestimate the power of your own intuition. When something feels wrong with you or a child, but the physician's response doesn't feel right, don't doubt yourself. Keep looking for answers and don't stop.

If I knew then what I knew how, I would've pushed even harder, even faster.

In order to sustain that push, it's vital to take care of your own mental and emotional health too. Severe illness can result in tunnel vision. Everyone focuses on the crisis, the fire that has to be put out. But don't forget about the other members of your family who are dealing with this too. Make sure everyone's feelings have been processed, so there are not lasting residual emotions that can damage relationships.

As a practical matter, finding doctors who are nearby or who allow you to do treatments in the home is a game changer.

I can attest that traveling to doctors when you or your child is sick will run you ragged very quickly.

Look for a doctor who can help coordinate and mediate between the other doctors, as Dr. Kaplan has done for us, if you can. Having to interpret, as a nonmedical person, what the physicians are saying or doing can be exasperating. It's not easy to find, but for us, spending a little more money for a doctor like this made all the difference.

And remember, most people who have changed the world and done impactful things have suffered trauma, tragedy, or incredible strife in their lives. As a result, they know the depth of their own personal power in a way that many adults never discover. You don't have to enjoy the struggle to appreciate the value of this knowledge.

We are used to things happening at lightning speed today, so it's getting harder and harder to wait. But keep in mind that even with the best outcome, it could be years before the situation gets better. For our family, it was painstakingly slow, but we got there.

Illness can be socially and emotionally isolating. Most people can't relate. Don't expect them to. This experience will change you in ways you can't anticipate. Hang onto the people who can hang in there with it.

Going through something not well understood, I really would implore physicians to remember that what isn't true or hasn't been discovered yet today may be true tomorrow.

We never faulted them for not knowing the answers. But we felt betrayed when they weren't even curious scientifically. Giving up on a patient who is suffering is the worst thing a medical professional could do. Not having the answers is fine. Not being willing to think outside the box or wondering what else we could do is a real disservice to suffering patients.

Continuing to ask "What else can I try? What else is out there?" is extremely important. Dr. Gary Kaplan and the people in his practice are truly curious and patient-centered and that makes all the difference, not only in the process but also, I daresay the outcomes.

There's a lot of shame in illness and people don't want to hear about it, but get out there. There are others out there. If you can help someone else and build the human connection that is so lost these days, then the journey you take is not alone and not in vain.

TREATING SARAH

DIAGNOSES

- Lyme and tick infection
- Mold toxicity
- Psychological issues
- Autoimmune Encephalopathy (POTS/PANDAS)
- Chronic inflammatory demyelinating polyneuropathy (CIDP)

First, we have to restructure our understanding of what the problem is, then what we test for, and then how we treat it. You can work with your doctor to encourage this perspective.

In Sarah's case, an autoimmune reaction was tripped off by all the tick-borne infections she had. We eliminated those first, then treated the autoimmune encephalopathy (POTS/PANDAS). When old symptoms remained or new ones flared up because her immune system was in a heightened state of inflammation, we looked for and identified other contributing factors: mold toxicity and psychological issues.

OUTCOME

Sarah is currently back in high school, full-time. She is a fearless athlete who was initially a "flyer" for her cheerleading squad and has grown into a strong, beautiful young woman who will be part of the base on her team this year. She has a great group of friends and is active socially. She still needs to be careful about mold exposure. Some days are hard. She is still in counseling because the years of illness took their toll, but with therapy she is coming to terms with understanding just how sick she was and what it is taking to reclaim her life. The family is also undergoing readjustment. When a child has been as sick as Sarah, your life has been surging from one crisis to the next. Fortunately, everyone is healing, and Sarah's future is bright.

LISTENING

If you have high blood pressure, a urinary infection, or a strep infection, the medical solutions are pretty straightforward. We have a pill for that. We also have an insurance system that rewards simplicity and penalizes, or – as Sarah's mother might argue – *punishes* complexity.

If you have a condition that can be diagnosed and treated within the 15 minutes of face time for which the insurance system will reimburse your physician, you can get the benefit of that reward. Your physician, however, will not be sharing that reward, since he will never be reimbursed for the additional 15 minutes he must spend documenting your visit. Time is money in the insurance system, and the whip-cracking enforcement with which that particular corporate overlord metes out penalties makes it clear that that it does not consider your physician's time to be worth much.

While you wrangle with your health, argue with your insurance company, and bemoan the skyrocketing costs of decent medical care, your physician engages in a parallel battle as the medical provider. Whether or not he or she is devoted to providing you with the best care possible, the sad reality is that the amount and quality of time your physician spends with you is largely dictated by what the insurance system will pay for – not by what you need for a comprehensive diagnosis and treatment.

Complex medical conditions require time. Time to listen to what is frequently an extensive and sometimes bizarre-sounding medical history is the single most important part of any medical visit. Time to do a thorough exam and run the appropriate tests is also essential. They also require time to reflect on the complexities, explore the medical literature, pursue tentative theories and educated guesses, and then follow up to confirm. This is absolutely imperative.

In my practice, I specialize in the complex conditions. After offering my best insights into the nature of these conditions in my first book, *Total Recovery*, I began to get patients who suffered from a far greater level of complexity. What I had thought were complex cases appeared relatively straightforward compared to these new conditions.

You don't have to be alive very long to realized that life has a perverse sense of humor. Once you think you've figured things out, it's only a matter of time before everything you thought you knew is thrown into doubt.

In this case, what I thought I understood about the immune system and the brain was a good start, but only a fraction of the whole story. Medical science is about coming up with a theory about how something works, then testing it to see if holds up under different situations. When the facts don't match the theory, you have to change the theory.

One of the things I love about my profession is that it constantly leaves me humbled and in awe of the natural complexity of the human experience.

STRANGE SYMPTOMS

By the time I saw Sarah, I had already started to hear strange stories at medical conferences from physicians whose work I respected about patients with seemingly bizarre symptoms. When they showed up as case reports in the mainstream medical literature, they were, for the most part, dismissed as psychiatric problems. The lack of comprehension was so entrenched that it had even descended into ridicule toward treating physicians for thinking these could be anything other than psychiatric cases.

It might have been no more than a source of mild, peripheral interest for me, except that more and more, I was starting to hear similar stories from patients: complaints of strange noises, transient episodes of blindness, multiple daily losses of consciousness, and total body paralysis.

When the neurologic testing and evaluations came back normal, the natural reaction of a mainstream physician is to make a quick referral to a psychiatrist and get the hell out of dodge.

Again, had the story ended there, I might never have pursued it, but most of the patients who were evaluated by psychiatrists were told they were not crazy. There was clearly a physical cause for their bizarre experiences. Almost overnight, they had become seriously disabled, unable to attend school, to hold down jobs, or interact with friends and family to a degree that caused a severe crisis in their lives. But the cause was medical, so the psychiatrists did not have anything to offer.

As these patients began to trickle into my clinic, they carried an additional burden: their profound discouragement over the months and years they'd spent being evaluated at some of the best medical centers in the country only to be told bluntly that there was nothing that could be done for them.

DOGMA OVER FACTS

An accomplished and intelligent woman, Sarah's mother was particularly appalled by the lack of curiosity in the scores of physicians Sarah had seen. Quick to dismiss her symptoms the moment they did not fit cleanly into a textbook classification, they blindly placed dogma over facts.

Although they must have felt that their adherence to premade categories they'd learned in their medical school or residency made them better physicians, the decision to override the facts in front of them was closer to religious fanaticism than medical science.

They might have suspected as much had they remembered the remark of Galileo Galilei, the brilliant Italian mathematician, physicist, and philosopher, who, when forced by the church to recant his finding that the Earth moves around the sun, responded, *"Eppur si muove."* ("And yet it moves.")

BELL'S PALSY

Sarah's initial symptoms looked like Bell's palsy, which causes weakness of the muscles of one side of the face due to damage to the facial nerve. One side of the mouth muscles stop working, resulting in a crooked smile, a tendency to drool, sensitivity to noise, and even ear pain.

These are only symptoms, not the disease. When the disease is caused by a virus, it typically resolves on its own with no special treatment other than supportive care. When it is caused by Lyme disease, it will not resolve without treatment. It can damage the nerves in the face and head that control eye movement. Patients often begin to see double once that nerve is damaged.

Because the most common textbook cause of Bell's palsy is a virus, none of the physicians tested her for Lyme disease. And for Sarah, that was the root cause.

PANDAS

In late 1990s, Dr. Susan Swedo at National Institutes of Health began to publish papers linking a common throat infection caused by strep throat (which doctors refer to as group A beta-hemolytic streptococcal bacteria) to the sudden development of bizarre behavioral and psychiatric symptoms in children, such as obsessive-compulsive disorder and repetitive type muscle spasms. Dr. Swedo designated this condition "pediatric autoimmune neuropsychiatric disorders associated with streptococcal infection." The unwieldy name was quickly abbreviated to PANDAS.[216]

The idea that an infection, especially one as common as strep, could cause psychiatric symptoms was not greeted with enthusiasm by the profession. Over 20 years later, despite being supported by a great deal of research, it is still dismissed as implausible by many physicians today. *Eppur si muove.*

In 2012, Dr. Swedo modified the definition of PANDAS to pediatric autoimmune neuropsychiatric disorder.[217] The new distinction separated the clinical presentation from the infection. Subsequent research has linked the onset of this constellation of symptoms to other infections, including flu, Epstein-Barr virus (mononucleosis), mycoplasma pneumonia,[218] and Lyme disease.

What Dr. Swedo and others have proposed is that one of these infections sets off an autoimmune reaction causing the body's immune system to attack the brain and nervous system. The resulting damage to the brain expresses itself in strange psychiatric and behavioral symptoms.

In my own practice, children with PANDAS have exhibited a range of symptoms, including rage attacks, pseudo seizures, severely regressive behavior, dangerous impulsive behavior, eating disorders, depression, anxiety disorders, and suicidal ideation.

In another chapter, I will discuss one of my teenage patients, a truly sweet, kind kid, who has done thousands of dollars of damage to his parents' house by kicking down doors, breaking mirrors, and other household items because of this disease. He had also developed a severe eating disorder, a relatively rare occurrence in a teenage boy.

Fortunately, PANDAS and the damage it causes to the body are reversible with a comprehensive treatment program.

INSIGHTS

As I began to see patients with more and more complex presentations, I was forced to dramatically expand my understanding of how the brain becomes inflamed and how all the different parts of the immune system are involved in this process. This was a critical realization.

The more we understand what has gone wrong in the body and provoked the illness, the better we can make sense out of the symptoms, ask the right questions, do the right tests, and get the right solutions to give patients their lives back.

CHAPTER 9

EMILY | NOTHING WOULD EVER BE THE SAME AGAIN

At 16, I got my first major diagnosis from Children's Hospital in Boston, one of the top-ranking pediatric hospitals in the United States. I was optimistic and eager to find a cure.

Doctors told me I had a genetic tissue disorder called Ehlers-Danlos syndrome and postural tachycardia syndrome (POTS), a nervous system disorder. They admitted that these diagnoses didn't match all my symptoms, but naming the problem conveniently allowed them to stop looking for explanations.

Before they could answer the questions that remained, I aged out of the children's hospital, and they sent me away.

It took a few years for me to grasp that my whole life had changed, and nothing was ever going to be the same. As my condition worsened, I started missing more and more school. Finally, I just dropped out of high school to relieve the pressure and hopelessness I felt with every missed day.

When I finally saw Dr. Gary Kaplan in 2016, one of the first things he did was take me off a lot of the drugs. Between medicating the pain and learning to disconnect myself from my body to protect myself from its suffering, I was so out of it that I hadn't even realized how sick I had become. Dr. Kaplan taught me how to listen and reconnect to my body.

After a series of tests, he diagnosed me with Lyme disease and started a treatment regimen of IV-antibiotics and IV-IG.

To tell you the truth, I didn't want to hear it. For years doctors had poked and prodded me, taking my blood, running endless tests, then trying to convince me I had some sort of genetic and nervous disorders that didn't quite fit. Now the new guy was saying it was all because of a tick?

For some reason, that felt like the final straw to me. It was a simpler diagnosis, but I had a much harder time accepting it. Now that I was more in touch with my feelings, I was starting to see how burned out I was on all of this.

But I hadn't yet learned not to say "yes" to everything the doctors say if they're genuinely trying to help you. And it's not like I had a better idea myself, so I continued the treatment. It was two long years before I was told I was "better." The Lyme was gone.

Except I didn't feel better. And I had been focused on nothing but my health for seven years.

It was time for a change. When the treatments stopped, I started to reclaim my life. I finally got my driver's license at the age of 22 and took a part-time job for the first time. It's hard to explain, but those two things gave me a tremendous sense of liberation. Before then, I felt like I couldn't point to anything in my life and say: "That's mine."

For so long, I'd lived at the mercy of my illness, sacrificing everything in the hopes of putting it behind me once-and-for-all, so I could finally live a normal life. But I'd come to the end of that road. Whether I wanted to or not, I just couldn't go any further. I needed something for myself, something to call my own. So, I decided to go for a balance between living and trying to find a cure. And in the meantime, I worked on learning to adapt to the level of health I had on any given day.

STANDING UP TO DOCTORS

In the beginning, I tacitly assumed that the doctors *knew what was best*. Over the years, I've come to realize that the truth is that most doctors are trying to *do their best*. The difference in those two things can be light years apart.

When this all started, I was just a teenager. The doctors assumed, as I did, that I ought to take their word as law and do whatever they said. Today I believe that even kids should have an active voice in their treatments. But I'm not a teenager anymore.

Now I know that when a doctor gives you the information and presents a treatment plan, they are just telling me my options. I don't have to do all of it or any of it. It's up to me as the patient to sort out what's right for me. The doctors may not understand that. Most of them assume they know what's best, as I once did. But that's okay. The choice is mine.

Even though I'm not the doctor, I know my body in a way that no one else can. If I don't speak up about what I think is best, if I don't defend my own intuition about my health, I'm not going to get the care I need.

Once I was able to find my voice and be more up front with Dr. Kaplan about what I wanted, the better the treatments became. As he confirmed, the more I share with him, the more he can help me. He's been very onboard with this approach, and I think more patients need to speak out.

Doctors aren't the be-all and end-all. They don't know every single thing. That's okay. But you know your body the best. They are experts in their fields, which gives them tremendous credibility. But if we start to revere them as authority figures and look to them for emotional validation or worry about offending them as if they were our parents, we've given them too much power.

What it comes down to is this: You have hired them to use their expertise to guide you and give you information. The decision as to what's working and what happens next is up to you.

STANDING UP TO YOURSELF

Keep in mind that it's okay to say "no" to yourself too. Somewhere we get the idea that if we're strong, we have to say "yes" to everything, but that's not true.

Looking back now, I can see that I was often trying to blast my way through, starting every new treatment regimen so intensely, as if I were trying to prove to myself I could handle any pain and discomfort that came along. Maybe so, maybe not. But it's not always a good thing to try. Sometimes, it's a really bad thing.

Now I know better. I listen to my body during treatments. If a treatment is too much, I say so. It's not a sign of weakness at all. One thing I've learned is that not listening to your body is worse. It can cause a lot of damage. It's taken me a long time to be able to say that and not think I'm weak, or that I should be able to handle more, or that I've failed.

When I was diagnosed with Lyme disease, for example, I was put on three different antibiotics. It was very intense. You were supposed to gradually ramp up to full doses of all three, but I was very eager to ramp up quickly, so I did. "I don't care about the pain, side effects or symptoms," I told myself. "Put me in the hospital if you have to. I want to get better!" But within a month, I hit a wall and I still had 18 months to go!

I hadn't learned to look ahead and pace myself, so it was really hard on my body and not at all good for my health. You can brute force your way through something in the short term, but for long-term problems, that sort of stubbornness will work against you every time. You can't rush through a treatment. Your disease doesn't care that you want to speed through it. It's going to take the amount of time it takes. Whatever amount of time it is, that's what your body needs.

It took a while, but once I adjusted my treatment plan to my needs, I found a path that worked better for me. Eventually, I found that going to see Dr. Kaplan every week was too much, so I pushed it up to every other week or every three weeks. That way, my life isn't all about my illness. I have the time and energy to go places or work a little and that means a lot to me.

When I have setbacks, I make time to let myself rest. Even after all these years, I still find that hard to do. It's a constant process of trying to make the right choices. When you're diagnosed with a chronic illness, you start questioning things you took for granted before: Can I go to dinner with friends? Will the energy I feel right now dissipate too quickly? If I go out tonight, will I pay for it tomorrow by being exhausted all day?

Sometimes I've said "no" to more stuff than I needed to, because of all the times I said "yes" and paid the price afterward. I try not to regret those choices. I know it doesn't mean I failed to do it right, but that there is no right. No one can perfectly anticipate the outcome of every choice. The best we can do is keep making adjustments and learning as we go.

If it's hard for me to know what to expect with chronic illness, it's even harder for other people. My ability to do something changes so quickly. The sudden drop in energy or increase in pain requires me to keep from losing patience with myself, but it also takes a lot of patience from the people around me – especially when I don't always look sick.

With an invisible illness, people tend to say dismissive things like, "You look fine!" Or, "Oh, you're too young to be sick!" But even if I looked pale and ashen or had to rely on a wheelchair to get around, it would still be a challenge for others. Illness frightens people and makes them uncomfortable. They want to say the right thing without giving offense, but they don't know what to say. Offering to help can be misconstrued as patronizing but failing to help can seem cold-hearted. Even those with the best intentions can really get it wrong. I try to be understanding and remember I don't always get it right myself. It's a struggle for all of us.

If I can't cope with it gracefully, how can I expect other people to always know the right thing to do or say?

FRIENDS AND CARING

That's why it makes such a huge difference to have befriended other patients at The Kaplan Center. Over the years, we've become really good friends.

It makes a world of difference to talk to friends who know what it's like to live with chronic illness. As sympathetic as my family and other friends are, they simply can't understand the way someone can who's experienced it themselves.

That's okay, but there's a different level of closeness. Since we share a common language and experience, it also takes less energy to be around people who are also sick. We have shorthand with each other.

We do regular video conference calls together, since a lot of us live out of state. Whenever we're in town, we get together if we can. I've spent a lot of time with some of them.

Making these dear friends was an unexpected part of being a patient at The Kaplan Center, but it has been a huge, important part of my treatment. Instead of feeling like an isolated patient, struggling alone, I feel connected to the other patients and the staff, who have known me for a long time now. Trust has built up among us. I feel looked out for and cared for in a very personal way.

HOW THINGS ARE NOW

My energy, pain, and cognitive issues are the ones that most affect my ability to do things. The quality of my sleep is very poor. I never wake up rested.

Memory and focus are huge daily struggles. Despite the treatments, things are still not right for me cognitively. I can't pick up a book, read it, and remember what I read. Over the years, I've increased the number of books I've read, but I still have to re-read as I go, and I struggle to remember them afterward.

On top of that, the headaches and migraines are still a big thing. I always have pain throughout my body and very poor strength, so my stamina for standing and walking is still pretty low.

Have I gotten any better?

If I look at it in terms of pain and symptoms, it's hard to see any progress. Some things are better, but other things are worse. It's hard to compare year-by-year, since things have changed so much, and I've even added new symptoms now.

To see improvements, I have to look at my quality of life: how often I leave the house, how much independence I have now. In those important areas, there has been a huge improvement.

Overall, I'm more active and better functioning. I'm not as house bound.

My health is not any better, but my quality of life is better.

The biggest change for me is that my goals for my health are different than before. As it turns out, some of these symptoms are going to be chronic. Despite some of the smartest doctors giving it their best shot, no one's been able to eliminate them yet. And rather than pumping up my stress hormones and waging a constant fruitless battle against that reality, I've decided to go for acceptance.

I'll always have some of this stuff. So, I'm giving myself a break, letting myself know that I don't have to reach the goal of being perfectly fine. My goal is to regain a quality of life that I'm happy with. The real world is messy and uncomfortable for us all. And I'm okay with that.

TREATING EMILY

DIAGNOSES
- Lyme disease and other tick-borne diseases
- Ehlers-Danlos syndrome (Hypermobile type EDS)
- Autoimmune Encephalopathy
- Postural orthostatic tachycardic syndrome (POTS)
- Chronic inflammatory demyelinating polyneuropathy

The key, again, is to remain open-minded. It helps to develop a tolerance for uncertainty. Only when you let go of what you assumed you knew for certain can you find new answers.

In Emily's case, her autoimmune encephalopathy was tripped off by the Lyme infection, but she also experienced a host of symptoms, including sleep disturbances, fatigue, night sweats, shortness of breath, generalized pain, brain fog, leg numbness, and muscle weakness. We treated the Lyme, then focused on POTS to get the best results.

OUTCOME

Today, Emily is driving, working part-time and rock climbing, and has completed her GED. We are discussing plans for her to start college classes. Her desire to start rock climbing was fascinating because it came out in a session we were having on goals. The rock climbing was about reclaiming her confidence in her body and herself. She is well on her way to doing both.

Being sick as long as she has been really challenged her confidence in herself, but the reality is she is very bright and insightful and has a wicked dry sense of humor. One of the challenges with patients such as Emily is the assumption that all her symptoms can be explained by the EDS and POTS diagnosis. The problem is that we then stop looking.

In Emily's case, there were other issues and finding them has made all the difference. Lyme and other tick-borne illness were also a problem for Emily. The challenge has been to methodically address all of her issues. Emily's case is especially complicated, but with our new understanding of the persister forms of Lyme, she is on a treatment protocol to do away with Lyme disease once and for all. Because of the Lyme and the autoimmunity, she developed nerve damage to her peripheral nerves, which unfortunately has not been responsive to therapy. We are considering other options, but this particular form of autoimmune damage is hard to fix. There are reports of stem cell therapies or exosomes that might be helpful, but all of this is in the experimental phase.

We are also exploring the theory that in people with EDS, because of the hypermobility of their spine, there is a constant instability that results in an ongoing irritation to the spinal cord that may contribute to their pain. In Emily, we have been using regenerative therapies, an approach where we inject substances to improve the strength of the tendons and ligaments in her neck and upper back that improve the stability of her spine. The injections are administered under fluoroscopic guidance and are quick and safe. This approach has been very productive for a number of our EDS patients in reducing both their headaches and overall pain.

Medicine is evolving rapidly, and we are hopeful that by the publication of this book a whole new group of therapies will have proven themselves to be useful.

MISSED CONDITIONS

Once, years ago at Cirque du Soleil, my wife and I sat rapt as the spotlight focused on a figure perched atop a dauntingly high pedestal. A first we perceived it as a work of art, some type of sculpture, until it began to move, wrapping back-and-forth on itself like a living Mobius strip. With a series of snake-like movements, it gracefully unwound to reveal, not an inanimate object but a human being.

The male performer twisted and turned himself into positions that are impossible for the majority of us. It was as if he did not have a single bone in his body, as if none of his joints were connected. For me, as a doctor, his performance was fascinating and deeply disturbing. Any contortionist is flexible, by definition, but some people are *too flexible*.

Even from our seats in the stands, I could see that this level of flexibility could only be the result of a genetic disorder called Ehlers-Danlos syndrome (EDS). For those with EDS, the connective tissue that literally holds us together is broken.

While I had to admit that an exciting circus career as a contortionist was certainly a good way to put the condition to use, I also knew that this is a disease that cannot be left untreated. Super stretchable connective tissue ultimately results in painful joint dislocation and increasingly hyperflexible skin. When that hyper-flexibility extends to heart valves and arteries, as it does in certain subtypes of EDS, fortunately not Emily's, valves and blood vessels can rupture, resulting in a stroke or death.

I am astonished by how often this diagnosis is missed. EDS affects as many as one in 5,000 people.[219, 220] Of the 13 subtypes of EDS, by far the most common expression is hypermobility. While we know the genetics of all the other subtypes, we still do not know the genetics of the hypermobility type (h-EDS).[221] The Beighton Scale in the Appendix is a quick, easy test for h-EDS that assesses levels of flexibility. When Emily took the test, she ranked at nine, the highest possible score.

By five years old, Emily had already suffered four dislocations of her elbow. Her parents, and Emily for that matter, reported that she was a "clumsy" child always getting injured, and by middle school had sustained three concussions. Headaches began in childhood and became progressively worse as she got older. Nausea was a constant issue since she was in grade school, as was chronic pain and progressive fatigue. Lightheadedness and episodes of briefly passing out were also becoming a significant problem in grade school. Reading made the headaches worse, and she was missing more and more school because of her medical issues. By the time Emily reached sophomore year in high school, it was all just too much, and she had to drop out of school.

The first time I saw a child with EDS was during my medical training. The child was five or six years old and had sustained an injury that raised immediate concerns about child abuse. The history looking back was not all that much different than Emily's, and fortunately the brilliant pediatrician with whom I was training with at the time recognized that the child had EDS.

Because kids with EDS have loose joints, they tend to fall and injure themselves. Also, because the connective tissue holding their joints together is too loose, they very frequently dislocate joints. If you add POTS to the equation, falls and injury are the rule not the exception. Parents are too frequently accused of child abuse toward these children when nothing could be further from the truth. As with Emily's parents, they are attentive, loving, and very concerned about a child that is getting progressively sicker and disabled. Because physicians frequently miss the diagnosis, they do not get the care, guidance, and respect from the medical profession they need and deserve.

Chronic generalized pain is very common in people with hypermobile EDS. (It is estimated that at least 50 percent, but perhaps as many as 89 percent of people with EDS experience this pain.[222] The diagnosis of hypermobile EDS is all too frequently missed. It's reported to take up to 10–20 years to get a diagnosis. It is not uncommon for people suffering from this condition to remain undiagnosed until their forties.[223]

I once consulted on a case where a young woman had been diagnosed with fibromyalgia. She also had a history "being somewhat of a klutz" with frequent falls and sprains. As I inquired further, I learned that she had also suffered several joint dislocations from playing sports. Everyone, including the numerous doctors and her mother who was a pediatrician, had treated her fibromyalgia, dismissing these incidents as klutziness or just bad luck. She had h-EDS.

WHEN I GET UP, I FALL DOWN

The other very common problem related to hypermobile EDS is postural orthostatic hypotension (POTS). Most people (63 to 78 percent) with hypermobile EDS have POTS.[224] It causes fatigue, problems with digestion, and temperature regulation issues, as well as an unsettling tendency to fall down.

Any time we change positions, our bodies adjust the tension in our blood vessels, so our blood supply stays evenly distributed, thanks to our autonomic nervous systems.

The autonomic nervous system itself is divided into two parts: fight or flight (the sympathetic nervous system) and rest and digest (the parasympathetic system). These two systems constantly work to keep each other in balance. When things go wrong and the fight-or-flight part of your nervous system isn't working, it leaves you constantly in rest-and-digest mode. When the bear comes to get you, you end up as lunch.

With POTS, the autonomic nervous system does not stay balanced. It fails to tighten the blood vessels to the legs, so when the legs move, it impairs the flow of blood to the brain. The heart is then driven into overdrive, racing to pump the blood pooled in your legs to your brain and causing the light-headedness that makes people with POTS inclined to briefly pass out and fall down.

Doctors refer to this series of events by the fancy name *dysautonomia.*

For Emily, knowing her diagnosis included hypermobile EDS and POTS was important, but it was not enough. She was still so sick that she had to drop out of high school. In her own words, "They admitted that these diagnoses didn't match all my symptoms, but naming the problem conveniently allowed them to stop looking for explanations."

Unexplained by hypermobile EDS and POTS were the loss of feeling and muscle weakness in her legs, the sleep disturbances that left her exhausted all day long, the night sweats, and the episodes of shortness of breath. While her generalized pain, more severe fatigue, and brain fog are certainly seen in people with hypermobile EDS, the other symptoms were not a fit. Seeing Emily's condition from the perspective of an inflammation in her nervous system allowed us to ask a different set of questions and find better answers.

We tested Emily for Lyme and the results came back positive for a Lyme officially called Borrelia burgdorferi. She also had Babesia, a parasite carried by ticks that is one of the co-infections frequently seen in people infected with Lyme disease. With the discovery of the Babesia, her night sweats and sense of never getting enough air (air-hunger) now made sense.

LYME

While it is critical to get rapidly diagnosed and treated, only 80 percent of people diagnosed and treated early are easily cured. Unfortunately, about 10 to 20 percent of people go on to develop post-treatment Lyme syndrome or chronic Lyme.[225]

The most common symptoms of post-treatment Lyme are fatigue, joint pains that move around the body, muscle pains, neck stiffness, headaches, sleeplessness, irritability, and difficulty with memory, concentration, and finding words.[226] As a result, many people with this condition are told they have chronic fatigue syndrome or fibromyalgia instead. Country singer Kris Kristofferson was first diagnosed with fibromyalgia, then Alzheimer's, before being correctly diagnosed and treated for Lyme.

On the other hand, due to Lyme's suppression of the immune system, it is not uncommon to see a re-emergence of multitude of other issues keeping people sick: viral infections such as mono (EBV), CMV, or HHV-6. In addition, many people also suffer with mold toxins, yeast, and bacterial overgrowth resulting in leaky gut and poisoning by heavy metals such as lead and mercury. All of these issues need to be considered in people who continue to be sick despite their treatment for Lyme.

It doesn't help that Lyme uses a wide range of methods to avoid being destroyed by our immune system. In the process, it can trick the immune system into attacking our own tissue.

Although the diagnosis and treatment of Lyme today is extremely controversial, that is the salient factor to our discussion: Lyme diseases can cause our body's immune system to turn on itself, often provoking autoimmune encephalopathy.

WHAT YOU NEED TO KNOW ABOUT LYME

Diagnosis is often missed. Unless you happen to develop a bull's eye rash, your physician may not even think about the diagnosis.

Accuracy of the test is limited. If you are tested for Lyme within the first three weeks after infection, the test is only accurate 29 to 40 percent of the time. The CDC cautions that testing may not be positive for up to six weeks after infection.[227]

Misdiagnosis is common. Lyme disease has been called the "Grand Imitator." Many people are mistakenly diagnosed with chronic fatigue syndrome, fibromyalgia, multiple sclerosis, depression, or dementia.[228]

Co-infections are usually present. Infections by other diseases carried by the same tick are the rule rather than the exception.[229] Babesia, Bartonella, Ehrlichia, as well as other borrelia species like miyamotoi, frequently go untested and are missed.[230]

Lyme can hide. When Lyme disease has been partially treated with antibiotics, the tests may come back negative even though you still have the disease. Lyme can cause the immune system to become suppressed, which allows the bug to persist.[231] In this "persister" phase, it burrows deep into the tissue, slowing its rate of reproduction to avoid being killed by antibiotics. This has made it very hard to kill, but two old medications, dapsone and disulfiram, are proving themselves to be effective against this persister form of Lyme.[232]

The idea that Lyme and a range of other infections can cause our immune system to attack itself is a fairly new concept.

Emily had Lyme and other tick-borne infections, but the infections had caused her immune system to malfunction. The path forward required treating the infections and her immune system as well as managing her hypermobile EDS.

TESTS THAT DON'T HELP

The standard tests for diagnosing the classical autoimmune diseases, like rheumatoid arthritis or systemic lupus erythematosus (SLE), will not reveal the diagnosis.

In her book *Brain On Fire*, Susannah Cahalan describes the horror of nearly dying from a newly discovered autoimmune disorder attacking her brain. She says a million dollars' worth of medical testing insisted she was healthy.[233]

All of my patients can attest to spending a lot of money on the wrong tests only to be told they were healthy when they were clearly very sick.

There are several consequences to this problem. First and foremost, you are still very sick without a path forward. Emily was so sick she had to drop out of high school. Her friends went on to learn to drive, graduate, attend college, and start graduate school or careers. She had a very close, loving family, but being this sick was still very isolating and frightening.

Second, the costs of being sick mount. Being this sick is very expensive, and insurance is increasingly unwilling to pay for testing. The average office visit is eight minutes. It is increasingly difficult to find a physician who will take the time needed to help.

So how do we make the diagnosis of a sick immune system in people whose illnesses started with an infection? A number of recognized tests can be considered by your doctor. Frankly, most of these will come back normal. The reason to do these tests anyway is about being thorough. The diagnosis of autoimmune encephalopathy, especially those caused by an infection, is a new and evolving concept. We are still discovering new antibodies that attack different receptors in the brain. These people are very sick. The goal is to not overlook anything.

In Part IV, you will learn about the labs that are doing breakthrough testing for autoimmunity related to infections, so you can get the most accurate and useful tests yourself.

Many physicians still do not know about these tests. Knowing about them yourself will provide you with a path forward in working with your physician. For Emily, it is still baby steps. Emily was 100 percent disabled for years. She had to drop out of high school. She is now driving a car again for the first time in years. Indeed, she is now driving her first new car, a forest green Subaru. She had been working part-time in a coffee shop, but that ended with the pandemic. She wanted to go rock climbing and has done so both indoors and outdoors. She has been able to travel to visit friends on her own and was even able to take a trip to Puerto Rico with a friend. She has completed her GED and is now taking college classes. One of the things I have always admired about Emily is how strong-willed and determined she is. Pacing her recovery is the challenge now, so she does not move too fast and set her recovery back. That being said, she is a remarkable young woman who has the intelligence and mindset necessary to truly recover.

INSIGHTS

The first challenge is to get the right diagnosis. This requires breaking from the idea that one disease/condition can explain everything. Sometimes the picture is very complicated with a number of problems that can make the other problems worse.

The correct diagnosis will need to explain *all of your symptoms*, not just some. Getting the right diagnosis requires asking the right questions, taking a comprehensive history, and doing the right tests. If you are still sick, the right questions haven't been asked yet.

If the testing is normal, it is not your fault and it does not mean that you are crazy. Do not give up. These illnesses present unbelievable challenges as well as extraordinary psychological pressures. We will be addressing these emotional challenges and what you can do about them in the following chapter on how to get support.

—

CHAPTER 10

NATHAN | TERRIFYING PERSONALITY CHANGE

As told by his mother

n March 2014, when Nathan was 14, he got a high fever that lasted for days. Afterward, he was not the same. The change was dramatic.

We could barely recognize his behavior. Nathan had always been a happy kid, eager to go outdoors, but suddenly, he was crippled by anxiety and afraid to leave the house. Day after day, he refused to eat, while we watched him dwindle before our eyes. When we asked him to get on the scales, we saw he'd lost 40 pounds.

Always thoughtful and intelligent, Nathan was suddenly subject to raging meltdowns – shouting, throwing furniture, breaking things – after which he would frantically crawl under his own bed and hide. It was super scary.

We finally got in to see the doctors at Children's Hospital in July 2014. By that time, Nathan was a shell of his former self. When he didn't test positive for strep, they decided it was mental.

From Nathan

THE SCARIEST PART

At first it was almost like the weirdest thing I've ever experienced in my life. Suddenly, I was scared of everything, and I didn't know why. My body was in pain. I hated myself intensely, but again, I had no idea why. That was the scariest, the emotional part.

As his mother, I always knew Nathan was sick, not mentally ill, but I couldn't prove it. I called Dr. Kaplan.

I'd known him long before he was famous and in such demand, when you could easily get in to see him! Any time I had weird symptoms, I'd call him.

Years earlier, I'd had severe, intermittent pain in my ribs myself. I'd consulted six different doctors for it before I found Dr. Kaplan. One after another, they came up with diagnoses that were so far afield it was almost embarrassing ("It must be asthma!" All kinds of crazy stuff.)

The pain didn't let up, so I had to keep searching for answers, but I didn't actually expect a cure by the time I met with Dr. Kaplan. Then he examined me.

"It's not asthma," he said. "You just cracked the cartilage between your ribs." He gave me a shot and that fixed it.

Another time, I woke up with extreme vertigo and hearing loss. The doctors supposed I had Meniere's disease, a disorder of the inner ear. No one's quite sure what causes it. The list of speculations includes everything from fatigue to emotional distress to changes in barometric pressure to too much salt in your diet.

The symptoms were bad enough to bring my life to a halt. I'd be shopping in a store and have to call my mom to come get me, then lay down on the floor to keep the room from spinning until she got there!

I knew Dr. Kaplan did acupuncture, which was purported to help, so I made an appointment. On the second treatment, he said, "It's not Meniere's disease, it's TMJ." He sent me to a dentist who fixed it.

Dr. Kaplan is really good at figuring out things.

So, when everyone said Nathan was mentally ill and I knew he wasn't, I went to see him. When it comes to saving people's lives, people on the cutting edge like Dr. Kaplan are driving the bus.

His schedule was so busy that we couldn't get in for months, so in the meantime, we took Nathan to the Anxiety Center for daily therapy. No matter what we did to get him help, he kept deteriorating. Nothing helped.

The Anxiety Center decided he must have an eating disorder. I didn't think that could explain the bizarre symptoms he was having, but it was true he wasn't eating, so we had him evaluated by a residential eating disorder clinic. Unfortunately, they had no space for boys.

From Nathan
FORGOTTEN
Even now, a lot of these experiences are mixed together in my brain. I don't remember them clearly. I've lost memories of things. An entire year is missing!
All I remember is that my whole body was hurting, and I was miserable. Maybe I'm better off without those memories! I think about that a lot.

Next, I found an outpatient clinic an hour away in Columbia, Maryland. I drove Nathan there every day. He met with therapists privately and we all met with therapists as a family.

As with the whole eating disorder diagnosis, they looked for the easy answer. I'm a yoga teacher who is well-informed about the value of healthy eating. I don't buy junk food for my kids. I insist on serving a good combination of fresh, healthy foods at home. They decided that must be the problem: I was to blame. I was too controlling, too insistent about good nutrition. I knew it wasn't that.

Years later, the therapist at those meetings apologized to me for leaping to that glib conclusion when she didn't know what else was going on. I appreciated her candor, but it didn't change the fact that the experience wasted precious time while Nathan was getting worse. On Thanksgiving 2015, Dr. Kaplan saw Nathan, along with my husband and me. He listened to our description of Nathan's symptoms for three hours, asking thoughtful questions the whole time.

When we were finished, he said, "This is not mental illness. It's inflammation. If I can find the cause of inflammation, I can fix it."

After running a series of tests, Dr. Kaplan told us Nathan had Lyme disease. He put him on antibiotics and in three days, my kid was back!

From Nathan

THAT MEANS I CAN FIGHT

In my whole life, I'd never experienced mania. But during this time, I felt totally out of control. I remember that part really well. It was really scary.

It started off as an eating disorder mixed with a kind of body image problem I'd never had before mixed in with lots of violent, manic behavior. A few times I started hallucinating. I thought I was losing my mind. It's like I was glitching out of this world.

All kind of crazy stuff was racing around in my brain. I'd try to convince myself to ignore it, that it was just me, being crazy. At first it was something I said privately to myself, but then a lot of doctors at the hospitals started saying it. And that exacerbates it in a major way because you obsess about it, going in this circle: Am I crazy? Am I not? It pushes everything down the hill, rushing out of control. It makes you crazier.

The thing is, when you're going through it, you kind of know it's not just in your head. But these professional doctors are telling you differently, so at some point, you give up and think, Sure, okay. I'm crazy.

But then Dr. Kaplan, for some reason, had a completely different approach than most of the others. He ran more tests, blood work, all sorts of different stuff. There were these vitamin infusions that maybe helped, maybe not. But I'm here now. And he finally got us a diagnosis!

That was when I put on my Big Boy Coat. I was like, "okay, so it's not mental. I'm sick. That means I can choose to fight it."

I finally knew I wasn't insane. That's when my perspective changed, and I was able to be a lot more positive. I was so happy to have an answer, even though he said it was going take a long time and it was going to be hard. But then, I had no idea how painful it would be....

In February, Nathan was still on antibiotics, feeling much better overall, though not great. It was his tenth grade year in high school and he was only able to attend for five months.

After dramatically improving when we began the antibiotics, his health gradually began to slide. Then one day, he got really ill.

We were at a friend's funeral. Because Nathan had really been struggling, my mom stayed home with him while we went to the service, then brought him to the restaurant afterward. He was so tired that he lay his head in my lap the whole meal, something he hadn't done since he was a child. Then all of a sudden, he twitched as if he were falling asleep, but the twitching increased, building into alarming, full-blown convulsions.

When we couldn't shake him out of it, my dad simply threw him over his shoulder and took him to the car. We rushed to the nearest suburban emergency room. Soon, the doctors shared our alarm: the convulsions lasted more than 24 hours.

No medications worked. It looked like grand mal seizures, but the brain activity said otherwise. Even when they transferred him to Children's Hospital, no one could stop the convulsions. When they finally stopped on their own, Nathan couldn't walk.

A week later, I took him home in a wheelchair. The infectious disease experts were resigned. "It's post-Lyme syndrome. There's nothing we can do."

I couldn't accept that. "It's an infection," I argued. "*Of course*, there's something you can do! You expect me to take my 15-year-old son home in a wheelchair and say that that's his fate? I don't think so!"

That day I hated the infectious disease people at Children's. They were relying on 25-year-old data and didn't know what they were talking about. If they couldn't even keep up with the research in their own specialty, how could I be expected to believe them?

From Nathan
OUT OF NOWHERE
It never seems to end. A lot of times we think we have it under control and then it comes back to me out of left field: all these convulsions start again.

Once we thought we had it completely under control for almost a full year, then I go to a rehab program in North Carolina. I have severe convulsions and end up in a wheelchair again! Totally unexpected and out of nowhere. That hangs over my head constantly, whether I like it or not, the possibility that it is still there. It's happened plenty of times in the past. You think you're safe, then it attacks.

It was like that in the early years when Nathan got sick. There were so few resources, so few medical experts who knew what was going on. In the last five years, so much has changed!

For one thing, Lyme disease wasn't as prevalent in the past as it is today. Not only was it misdiagnosed as something else, but the actual number of incidents has also gotten worse. According to the CDC, there were more than 12,000 cases of Lyme disease in 1997. Just 20 years later in 2017, it's estimated that there were more than 40,000.[234]

It's a stealth disease. Nathan was never aware of being bitten by a tick, but he always spent most of every day outside. We live on 2.5 acres of land in Darnestown. We hike together as a family. We love nature. Any one of us could've been bitten by ticks on countless occasions. Maybe we would have noticed it, maybe not.

When I first told people he had chronic Lyme disease four or five years ago, people didn't know about it. The standard treatment was to take antibiotics for ten days and you'd be fine. Now when I mention it, people immediately say they're so sorry. They realize how awful it can be. So many of their friends and neighbors have suffered from it too. That's a new reaction.

Now at Children's Hospital, there's a whole new protocol. Even in the emergency room, potential Lyme patients have to see a neurologist. It makes me feel so happy. I know I had a part in that change.

After Children's Hospital was content to leave Nathan in a wheelchair for life, we went to New York University Hospital for about a year and a half. It was a long commute back and forth. My mom made significant contributions to their work, even though I tried to talk her out of it. I thought it was insane to give them time and money, but she persevered.

But now they've built an Autoimmune Encephalitis Center with my mom's grant money.

It didn't happen nearly soon enough to spare Nathan and our family from years of misery, but as people became aware of the complexity and legitimacy of this diagnosis, things gradually began to change. It's heartening to see that happen at last.

As with any bureaucracy, it takes a while for them to catch up. For years, they stick to the CDC's outdated guidelines or the studies that have proven successful because that's how big institutions have to operate. Until they don't.

If Lyme disease were the only problem, we might have completely restored Nathan's health by now, but like Dr. Kaplan says, it's like peeling an onion.

Lyme is one layer. Then it became clear that he also has Bartonella, which I believe caused his convulsions. Beneath that is Babesia, then chronic Epstein-Barr. You eliminate one, it frees up room for the next one to flare up. As soon as they do, we call Dr. Kaplan, and he fights them back.

We owe so much to Dr. Kaplan. I love that man.

Yet, as much progress as we've made, we almost lost Nathan in January 2018.

Nathan had been open about the fact that he had been self-medicating with marijuana for the previous two years. Dr. Kaplan recommended that he stop, and when he couldn't, we sent him to a rehabilitation program in Asheville, North Carolina. It's beautiful country and Nathan has always been an athlete, so he couldn't resist going hiking on the weekend. It was a mistake.

After 16 days, the convulsions started, and they rushed him to the hospital. Nathan was in severe pain. He's always in pain, but somehow this was magnitudes greater. He'd have a convulsion, then wake up screaming at the top of his lungs, pass out, then stop breathing. Then the whole thing would start again. This went on for two whole days. It was terrifying.

Since I was in Miami taking a much-needed break, it took me 24 hours to reach him. I've never been so scared. He was having convulsions the whole time. Even today, his legs are still atrophied, and he's got severe neuropathy from the convulsions. For an athlete, that's especially hard.

The IV-IG helps. They did that in Asheville. Although he is allergic to certain brands, Gammagard works for him. And by a stroke of luck, they had it (Not all hospitals do. Children's Hospital, for instance, never carried it. We always had to wait for the special order to arrive.)

The number of relatively little things that have gone wrong every step of the way is countless, as anyone who's been through this kind of medical crisis knows. Sometimes I amaze myself with my ability to keep going despite it all. The experience has definitely changed me in a lot of ways. It's repeatedly forced me to do things I didn't even know I was capable of.

I'm a yoga teacher, not a yeller. But I've stood in ERs and screamed at doctors at the top of my lungs. At Children's Hospital, when Nathan's pediatrician called me and told me smugly that it wasn't Lyme, I started screaming at her, accusing her of spouting opinions though she was completely ignorant of the latest medical research. My husband applauded.

Today Nathan is 19. He hasn't been in a wheelchair since January 2018. He gets IV-IG every three weeks, and it helps. The anxiety issues have subsided enough that he doesn't need medication. He's off the antibiotics entirely. Last semester he took two classes and really enjoyed them.

At long last, we have a firm diagnosis: *Autoimmune encephalitis caused by tick-borne infection.*

He's doing so much better now. His quality of life has greatly improved. This summer, he got both his GED for high school graduation and his driver's license in the summer, finally. (I even trust him driving, which amazes me.) He's always had a girlfriend, but now that she goes to school in North Carolina, Nathan takes the train by himself to see her. He's still dealing with flare-ups from time to time, but he's finally the happy boy I recognize again, and he's a lot more independent than before.

For my own part, I'm cautiously optimistic. We've been in a space before where things looked better. I never forget that. But I try to live in the moments between crises, to accept every day on its own terms, and to not project my own fears or worries. I don't know what's going to happen. None of us do.

As a family, we're a lot calmer now in a crisis. We can even laugh about it while it's going on sometimes. People would probably think we're insane. Even Nathan can laugh between convulsions, when the whole thing's too absurd to be believed.

It's not that we're not as caught up in it. We are. When a crisis hits, it has our full attention. More than 100 percent, I'd say. But the magnitude of those crises has taught us not to get as caught up in the trivial things. That part of it is a real gift.

We see people around us worrying all the time about things we can't even be bothered to worry about anymore. We used to do it, too, of course; it's normal. But now there simply isn't time. It forces you to see the trivia for what it is and let it go. As a family, this has profoundly changed all of us. Nathan's the same way. When his friends are complaining about a big test, he doesn't get caught up in it.

From Nathan
HOW IT WAS BEFORE
It's true, it changes you. I have these worries, but because I have these worries, I don't worry about anything. Interesting phenomenon.

I've also noticed that the level of what causes me to panic is much higher than the average person's.

When I was younger, some little glitch might come up and derail me and my mom for a full day. We'd go to music practice and the sheet music would be missing or the teacher would be late, and it would bend us all out of shape. We'd be telling my dad about it over dinner, totally derailed. There's no way that would derail us now.

When Nathan decided to take the SAT, he signed up and then told us. Five days later, he showed up. He just went. He never opened a book or researched it, so he didn't even know you needed a calculator. When he realized it, he just took it without a calculator. As it turned out, he didn't have the stamina to make it through the test, yet he did really well on it – a higher than average score. Now he's doing it right, taking an SAT class, doing the preparation. He knows he can do better and is motivated to take it again. But I love that he just went. The boldness, after all he's been through, inspired me. I can't count how many times he's been knocked down, brutally hard, but he's always gotten up again. He doesn't see the limits. I admire that.

From Nathan
THE THING YOU CAN'T SEE

I'm just glad to not be in constant neurological pain every day. That's the biggest difference in my life now. After a lot of infusions, my body's hemoglobin and my immune system got stronger, and it finally went away.

Before that, I used to have the daily sensation of someone setting loose armies of ants inside my body, then lighting them on fire. I could feel them crawling around beneath my skin, really hot, constantly. It was such a distracting, painful sensation that it would really mess with my brain. I'm so glad it's gone. Even thinking about it makes me cringe!

It started suddenly one day after a convulsion. When I came out of it, I couldn't use my legs and that sensation started. Eventually I could use my legs. But that horrible, crawling-burning sensation didn't go away for years.

It's hard for people to understand without experiencing it, but that crawling-burning thing was actually far worse than not being able to use my legs. It's constant torture. It keeps you up at night. And it makes you irritable. People meant well, when they looked sadly at my legs and felt bad for me. But I couldn't feel my legs anyway! They didn't bother me. They weren't in pain. What was really driving me crazy was the thing they couldn't see.

A lot of times, things we can't see are the biggest things people are dealing with.

I knew it wasn't their fault. And I never really told them because I didn't want their sympathy, but it really taught me something. We have no idea what people are dealing with.

TREATING NATHAN

DIAGNOSES

- Lyme and other tick infections
- Autoimmune Encephalopathy

In Nathan's case, he had several tick-borne diseases that we needed to treat first, then we had to fix the gut. The intestines are not only critical for healthy nutrition but are also a critical part of your immune system. In Nathan's case, both the innate and acquired immune systems needed to be repaired. So, antibiotics, nutrition, supplements, and IV-IG were crucial for his recovery.

Therapy is also frequently a necessary part of recovery. Patients and their families have been traumatized by the illness and not infrequently by the medical profession and fighting battles with insurance companies that do not want to pay the medical bills. Their lives have been upended, and support is necessary to help make sense of what has happened, regain their confidence, and reengage in life with confidence.

Nathan was very sick, terrifyingly so. Crippling anxiety, rage attacks, distorted body image (*body dysmorphia*), and 40-pound weight loss from an eating disorder were his symptoms. A brief episode of strep infection was gone when he was first seen by a physician at Children's Hospital, one of the leading hospitals in the country. With such dramatic psychological presentations, they shipped him off to a psychiatrist.

The very first order of business for anyone this sick is to make sure they are safe, so having him evaluated and treated by a psychiatrist was an important step. But it completely ignored his history and the very sudden onset of this extreme condition.

A month earlier, Nathan had been a happy and healthy teenager, not an inherently unstable or violent kid. Between his fits of rage, there was still a delightful sweetness about him. The very fact that he had always been such a gentle soul made these violent rages even more alarming.

Over the years he did thousands of dollars of damage, but it was telling that his violence was always directed at things (breaking furniture, doors, plates, glass windows) never toward hurting anyone – not people or animals.

On more than one occasion, his father had to literally wrestle him to the ground and prevent him from doing more damage or running away, as he was prone to do during these episodes. To his father's great credit, he always took the blows and never once hurt or injured Nathan.

Stress always triggered the outburst, though it was not necessarily something that you, I, or even Nathan would normally regard as a big deal.

Each event would last a limited time, then Nathan would fall asleep, exhausted. To me this sounded like a seizure, but neurologic testing for seizures was normal. Whether or not it is related to autoimmune disease for any particular person, it can sometimes be helped by medication that helps calm the brain, such as lithium, SSRIs, non-steroidal anti-inflammatory medications (NSAIDs), and low-dose naltrexone.

When mental illness can be traced back to an infection that launched an autoimmune response, as in Nathan's case, our options are entirely different.

We were able to do the unthinkable with Nathan: cure his violent mental illness with antibiotics.

It worked because his sudden change in behavior was caused by an infection. We also found that when he eliminated his Lyme disease, his eating disorder disappeared.

This was not an overnight cure. There were multiple set-backs and a need to adjust the treatment as more infections were uncovered. This has taken several years of treatment. His own immune system was attacking his brain and he required, and still does require, ongoing treatment with Intravenous Immunoglobin. The rage attacks are gone, the pseudo sei-zures are gone, and the obsessive-compulsive behavior and eating disorder are gone. The delightful, thoughtful, and kind Nathan is back.

TIPS FROM NATHAN'S MOM

TRUST YOUR GUT. It sounds weird, but listen to your gut instinct. Too many people listen to their own mental chatter or whatever everybody else has to say, when they know in their gut what the best decision is. Trust your gut.

DON'T BLAME YOURSELF. When you're tempted, just remind yourself of that classic refrain about how point-lessly too late it is: *coulda woulda shoulda!*

WHAT WORKS CHANGES. Eating no sugar helps for a while, but then it doesn't. Certain herbs or supplements help, then they don't. But something starts to help. It's fluid. There's no one thing. I suppose it's because he had more than one illness, so it shifted. But who knows?

THE OTHER SIDE. Most people do come out the other side. If you expect things to get better, you tip the scales in that direction. There can be a huge healing impact in that belief. If you assume things are not going to get better, it's definitely harder to recover. You're stacking the deck against yourself. There is another side. You can't always see it, but just keep taking steps in that direction, even if you have to pretend you believe, and chances are you'll get there.

HACKS FROM NATHAN'S MOM

EPSON SALT BATHS. These help Nathan immensely. At his worst pain, he took four a day.

DETACH. In the moment, it's okay to create a little space. Imagine you are watching these surreal events in a movie. Put it on a screen. Take your emotional self out of it. For now.

PACK FOOD. We always bring food with us. I carry a cooler to the hospital, along with blankets and pillows for Nathan. Our go-to foods are healthy whole foods: fruit, cheese, seltzer water, and popcorn. We order UBER EATS in the hospital for at least one meal.

MEDITATE. As a yoga teacher, naturally I'm a big meditator. I don't know what I would do without my practice. It helps me stay calmer to breathe through things. When your kid is flipping out, it's easy to overreact. It's very scary, especially in the beginning, when you don't know if it's going to stop. It does stop, but for moment, you wonder if it's going to end. The calmer you can stay, the easier it is to find a creative solution to diffuse what could genuinely be a disaster.

BE THE ADULT. Your kid feels out of control. That's scary for them. If they're freaking out, it helps if you, as the adult, stay calm. Your calmness can directly prevent escalation. I've seen parents freak out and, believe me, it makes things so much worse for everybody.

SELF-CARE. This one is the hardest for me. There's so much to manage, so much to research, so much to worry about that it's easy to get into overdrive and not let go. It's important to find your own best ways to relax and do them no matter what. Personally, I tend to go hiking. Movement, stretching, or even just mindlessly watching some great new show on TV, also works. We binge-watch a lot with Nathan, especially things that make us laugh. We watch a lot of Netflix in the hospital when we're there for two or three days at a time for IV-IG. It makes a discernible difference. We're not as exhausted when we get home.

HACKS FROM NATHAN

EPSOM SALT BATHS. For me, for some reason, being in a warm bath is *pure*. It's the biggest relief I have. It's like an equalizer from the water on your body. Plus, I usually meditate to amplify the calm. Letting my brain flow really helps me relax. I can honestly feel it deflating and let my body un-inflame. I can almost picture it. That's been something I've been doing since I got sick. I never did it before. But it always makes me feel a lot better. It's definitely a hack.

DETACH. Your body comes up with its own toolbox of things you can do. Experience teaches you. I can't explain it, but when I was in the most pain, I learned how to detach from it. I called it *outside world* and *inside world*. Inside world was in my brain and whatever was happening to my body in outside world was separate from me. It made *a huge difference*. I did it all the time.

You can still feel the pain, of course, but it's not on you in the same way. You separate your emotions from the pain your body is experiencing to make it tolerable.

HAVE A "GO BAG." You never know how long a hospital stay will last and they really make you feel out of your element, so be sure to have a go bag ready with the stuff you like. Take your favorite blanket or pillow. We bring a cooler with my own specific foods. Since I kept getting extremely cold at random times when I shouldn't be cold, I'd take heat packs to put in my pockets. Jackets didn't help, but heat packs did. Don't neglect this one. Taking the things that work best for you can make the biggest difference in the world.

CHAPTER 11

—

JANET | KEEP LOOKING. I KNOW SOMETHING'S WRONG

was about five years old when I got bit by a tick. Apparently, it happened in upstate New York at summer camp. I never saw a rash but even at that young age, I started having headaches off and on. About a year later, my mom took me to my pediatrician, who found a circular rash on my head that should have told him it was a tick bite, but he must not have known what it was.

All through elementary school and middle school, I was in pain: first headaches, then back pain. Some days it was so bad that I would just lie on the floor. It seemed to be the only thing that even remotely helped. I really didn't know how to handle it. I missed a lot of school when I was a kid. But in high school, it got worse.

Thankfully, my parents believed me, regardless of other people's snide remarks about how I "just wanted to skip school" or I was "faking it."

The whole time, I kept pushing my parents to find answers. "Something's wrong," I said. "We need to find an answer!" I went from doctor to doctor to doctor. Each one put me on antibiotics and tried their own favorite medications, but nothing helped.

In high school, I was diagnosed with fibromyalgia, but I always considered that diagnosis to be more about their desire to name it than anything else. It's a broad, general diagnosis of pain in certain areas of the body. I thought, "Okay, I knew that. But *what's wrong!?*"

Eventually, every doctor got to a point where they said, "There's nothing more I can do for you."

There were no answers. Every single time I got my period, I was out for a week because the cramps were so severe I couldn't get off the couch.

My only option was to keep pushing through as best I could. I am very good at pushing through. I just put on a brave face and faked it.

NORMAL LIFE

In an effort to live a normal life, I went away to a four-year school right after high school like all my friends. But I didn't do well there. By the end of the first year, my parents said, "Come home, live with us, go to community college. We'll take care of stuff. You'll be fine."

In the fall of 2008, I enrolled in Burton Community College. I was still struggling with my illness, but the school offered special accommodations, like people to help me and take notes in class. It was just the kind of support I needed. Even though my brain was even foggier than before, it was just the support I needed to make it work. My grades were good.

I also learned that I needed to talk to my teachers to explain why I wasn't going to be able to make it to every single class. Some tied their grades to attendance, but when I explained, it typically went well. For two semesters, I was able to succeed at school. I signed up for a third semester, but by then my health was getting worse. I was continuing to see doctors, but they had no idea what to do for me.

Although writing had always come easily for me, I suddenly couldn't do it anymore. One day I was trying to write a paper and found that I was completely unable to put together any sentences whatsoever. I couldn't even brainstorm.

It felt like it was the last straw. I'd been struggling so much just to get to school. I'd always relied on my facility with writing to bring my grades up. It was the one thing that had allowed me to participate. With that gone, I knew. It was over. I had to drop out.

WORKING

If I couldn't go to college, I felt like I should try to do something else. The part-time job I took was a clear dead end. The number of hours I had to work to make any money was crazy. So, I went to bartending school.

My ability to sleep had become so unstable that I was awake all night anyway. I might as well work. Bartending school only lasted a few months and it turned out to be a good starting point.

After school, I got a job in a nightclub where I really started to flourish. My health was not any better, but I made a lot of money and really enjoyed myself there for a few years. I would wake up at 7:00 p.m., go to the club, and work until 3:00 a.m. In those few hours, I made more money than I'd made in a week in the previous job.

My health was so bad that work was the only thing I could do. Day after day, I was either sleeping or working. I was exhausted all the time, so I lived on Red Bull. But the great thing was that the place was usually packed, so I'd be moving nonstop all night with no time to think about how much pain I was in. Then the lights would come up and it was over.

I'd walk out to my car in the parking lot and crash. Many nights I was so sick I couldn't drive home. My parents would have to come out at 3.00 a.m. to take me home. I'd lie on the bathroom floor next to my mom and throw up.

"Why are you throwing up all the time?" She'd ask me, stroking my hair.

"I don't know, Mom," I'd tell her. And neither did anybody else.

LIMBO

For many years, I was in limbo, living in a haze of work and taking medication for the pain. I got my own apartment for a while and did the best I could to clean and cook, but I was so sick I can't even say now what medications I was on and which doctor I was seeing.

The stress and frustrations of what felt like a constant, futile struggle had resulted in a falling out with my parents, but my health took such a bad turn that they said, "Why don't you come home? We'll take care of you. You don't have to work. We'll just find another doctor and try again."

It's all very hazy after that, but by early 2012, my health started to spiral downward. Soon I was bedridden, relying on a wheelchair to get around. The pain and brain fog got much worse while my energy took a dive. When it got to the point that I couldn't feed or bathe myself, my parents hired a nurse caretaker who stayed with me all day while my mom was at work.

For my part, I just slept – sometimes for two or three days at a time. My mom feels like she should've woken me up more, but, honestly, I probably would've asked her to go away.

Just before we found Dr. Kaplan, I started having severe migraines that kept me from sleeping altogether. My nervous system became incredibly hyperactive. I developed such severe light and sound sensitivity and when my mom accidentally scraped a knife across a plate, it would send shockwaves across my body.

A doctor in New York state told me that IV infusions of a lipid called *phosphatidylcholine*, along with a high-fat diet would help. After all the IVs I'd been given over the years, my veins were shot, so they had to put in a port. And the high-fat diet made me gain weight.

Meanwhile, I was taking high doses of heavy-duty pain meds: Vicodin and Dilaudid. The pain management doctor said it was enough to knock out an elephant, but I barely felt a difference.

I told my mom, "We need to do something now. I'm spiraling so far out of control that I feel like I'm going to die." It felt like I had a very short window to make changes. Otherwise, I was going to be bedridden on a morphine drip for the rest of my life. What kind of life is that?

We took an emergency trip to a clinic in Germany for a week-long intensive of IVs, treatments, and injections. Afterward, my pain began to subside, and I felt my brain clear a bit, but all of it came rushing back when I got back home. It was as if the house itself was making things worse.

HOPE

By the time I finally saw Dr. Gary Kaplan, in March 2015, my port was infected, I was septic, and I had been suffering for as long as I could remember.

The only reason we heard about him at all was because one of my doctors had recommended his book, *Total Recovery*, saying, "You really should read this!"

I'd put my hope in so many doctors by this time that I didn't know if I could stand to be disappointed again. I was skeptical when I asked, "Do you think you can get me well?"

Dr. Kaplan immediately assured me, "I have a lot of tools in my toolkit, and I will try every single one."

If he'd said yes, it would've felt like another empty promise from a doctor who would ultimately shrug his shoulders and give up on me. But Dr. Kaplan didn't say yes. He said he'd try everything he possibly could. And that was enough for me. His candor allowed me to trust him.

KAPLAN CENTER INTENSIVES

At The Kaplan Center, Dr. Kaplan offers week-long intensives, too. I did it all: lymph drainage, cranial sacral work, visceral manipulation, acupuncture, psychotherapy. And I saw Dr. Kaplan every day for evaluation, along with prolotherapy and peripheral nerve therapy.

The intensives were really hard on me, but I'd go for one week every month. After each one, I'd feel better. For me, pro-lotherapy was extremely painful, but within a few months, the difference it made was amazing! For the first time, I felt like my treatments were making me progressively better.

One of the things Dr. Kaplan considers is environmental toxins. When he asked us to call in mold experts to investigate the possibility that our house had mold contamination, we did. The inspectors found a massive area of black mold behind my bedroom wall!

In no uncertain terms, Dr. Kaplan said, "Leave the house!"

I moved in with my grandma while my parents did the mold remediation. The previous owners had added on the two rooms where I lived, but they didn't do it properly. When the remediators opened the walls, they found layers of wallpaper over damp bricks and thick black mold. The room where I had been bedridden for so much of my life was riddled with mold!

Like many people, my body can't process mold toxins. When the genetic testing gave us proof, Dr. Kaplan put me on Cholestyramine and started a mold detox protocol.

With every new development, I could feel myself getting better.

TAKE A CLASS

Many of my symptoms had abated by the end of 2015, then I developed an incredible burning sensation in my legs. Dr. Kaplan prescribed Neurontin for the pain. To my surprise, it helped so significantly that I could stand up! Before long, I was actually able to start walking a bit.

When spring approached a few months later, Dr. Kaplan (who can be very demanding) said, "I want you to take a class!"

In our first interview, he had asked me, "What is your biggest fear?"

"Not getting well," I said.

"If you were well, what's the first thing you'd do?"

There was no question in my mind. "I'd sign up for classes."

When I first came to The Kaplan Center, I was in a wheelchair, and my mom had to help me out of that wheelchair. Now my pain had subsided enough that I could stand up on my own and take a few steps. Dr. Kaplan was right. It was time to take another kind of step.

I signed up for a world geography class online. Although my brain was clearer, I still needed my dad to read to me and help me write the essays. But it was really great to get back into school.

In the fall of 2016, I also started a three-week pain program at The Kaplan Center. It consisted of yoga, meditation, and nutritional education from 9.00 a.m. to 5.00 p.m. In the past, my mom had always stayed with me during the intensives. This time, she only came on the weekends. It was another encouraging step.

That month, the Positivity Journal I was keeping read:

Sept 19, 2016 - Walked to every appointment at The Kaplan Center.

Sept 20, 2016 - Left the wheelchair in the car.

I felt like I was getting my independence back. Then in January, the Lyme came back. I had to stop taking the world geography class because of the fatigue and pain. It was very disappointing.

Dr. Kaplan encouraged me to keep my hopes up. "Look how far you've come!" More than once, his attitude has allowed me to push forward, even when life pushes me back several steps.

FRIENDS AND TRAVELS

Around that time, Dr. Kaplan told me about the support group run by patients at the clinic. I'd been in support groups before, but I'd never liked them. This is different. Even though our symptoms aren't exactly the same, they're similar enough and the treatments are similar enough that it gives us a feeling of kinship.

It's been incredible to have these girls in my life. We do video calls every other week or so. I make a point to see any of the girls who are in town whenever I'm at the clinic. I believe it has made a tremendous difference in my mental and emotional health.

By May 2017, I was able to start driving again. It was an incredible moment of liberation. By summer, I was thriving: swimming every day in our backyard (sometimes multiple laps), walking every day (eventually more than a mile), journaling, and meditating. To my great delight, I even started reading *Game of Thrones*! My brain hadn't allowed me to read for a really long time.

After they dropped me off at The Kaplan Center in July, my parents went on a well-deserved vacation. While they were gone, I happily drove a rental car back and forth on my own.

That same summer, I spent a long weekend on the Outer Banks with my friend Joan. That was huge. It was the first time I did something away from my parents that wasn't medical!

We went to the beach, walked on the sand, went jet skiing and parasailing. I remember thinking, "Oh my god, my legs are not in pain!" I hadn't been to the beach in years because the burning in my legs was always excruciating. This felt like a normal vacation. I was over the moon.

Our time at the beach went so well that I flew to Florida the next month to visit my former nurse who had retired there. I went walking every day. When we went to Universal Studios, my device counted 23,000 steps that day. I was sore and exhausted, but free of leg pain and able to fly home. It was like a miracle.

COLLEGE FOR REAL

When fall rolled around, Dr. Kaplan was determined to build on my success. "A year from now, I want you in college full-time." I hadn't taken any classes that spring, but I took two in the fall and got As in both.

At first, my dad still had to read to me, but before long, I could read and write the essays myself. This was a big deal for me too. It felt like my writing ability, even though it wasn't quite as good as before, was coming back.

The college gave me academic forgiveness and my GPA rose enough that I could join the honor roll. Fairly quickly, I've worked my way back up to going to college full-time. I'm taking five classes and applying to four-year colleges. I'm out of the house most of the day at least four days a week. All of this is a really big deal for me.

We'll have to see what happens next. I hope I'll have enough energy to go away to school. I hope to attend college in Washington, D.C., and study international relations.

THE FUTURE

The biggest change of all is that I'm now able to look forward to a future for myself.

Of course, my optimism varies on any given day. It's always been my tendency to focus on what's wrong. When I do that, Dr. Kaplan brings me to Earth: "You're ridiculous. Just the fact that you're out of the house all day is amazing!"

"Yeah," I mutter, "but there are still some days when I come home and crash..."

There have always been peaks and valleys. Apparently, a lot of my valleys came from mold. Even after we eliminated the black mold from behind my bedroom wall, I was often exposed to unseen mold. I'd start to feel badly, Dr. Kaplan would test me for rising levels of mold toxins, and the tests would come back positive. Then the search would begin: Where was the mold hiding? One of those searches led to the discovery that there is mold behind the walls at the community college I attended.

The progress I've made since seeing Dr. Kaplan has been absolutely incredible. Any time I travel anywhere, I send him a postcard. Knowing that I have a heart for helping people all around the world, he recently said, "My dream for you is to send postcards from all the places you go around the world." That's my dream, too.

TREATING JANET

WHO IS SICK?

When I first met Janet, I asked her the same things I ask all my patients: "When was the last time you were in excellent health? When did you last you felt healthy, strong, and vital? What did your life look like when you were healthy?"

I also asked about her childhood and what kind of challenges she had faced growing up. It was important to know whether she had grown up in a nurturing, loving environment or one filled with significant emotional and physical challenges, because all of these things have a direct impact on the health and resilience of every patient.

The answers about health help me to understand what my patients have lost to their illness and what they believe is possible.

The answers about their formative years in childhood tell me about the terrain. We now know that significant socioeconomic deprivation and childhood trauma impact the immune system and significantly increase the risk of developing autoimmune disease as an adult. In fact, severe psychological stress impacts the actual structure and function of the mitochondria, the very powerhouse of our nerve cells in our brains.[235]

It is not enough to know what type of infection a patient has. It is also crucial to understand who is sick.

When I asked Janet about the last time she had been in excellent health, she could not recall. She had been sick for most of her entire life. Illness and disability were her baseline. No matter how many times or how valiantly she had tried to keep up with her peers, it had ended in terrible setbacks with her condition getting worse.

As if it were not enough to be forced to cope with a debilitating illness that no physician had identified, much less understood, Janet's home environment would have challenged the healthiest child. Her parents were loving and supportive, but their home life had always been chaotic at best.

It was a shaky foundation from which to deal with a chronic illness that always puts stress on emotional, physical, and financial resources. Feelings of hopelessness and helplessness about the situation can infect loved ones. It is not just the patient who is suffering, but the entire family.

Far too often, professionals make things worse by giving contradictory advice and offering hope that ends in disappointment.

Over time, Janet's world had shrunk to the size of her bedroom. In constant pain and crushing fatigue to the point of not being able to bathe herself, she required care 24/7. Only her capacity for withstanding this level of helplessness and dependency allowed her to survive.

ILLNESS IS A PROCESS

Studies have shown that three things allow us to adapt to adverse conditions: a sense of personal control over our lives, a positive attitude, and social support. Together, these things favor both psychological resilience and immunological resilience.[236]

Losing these things rarely happens all at once. A state depleted of psychological and immunological resources tends to evolve over time. It is a process, not an event.

As we have said, infections can ignite a fire that builds into autoimmunity.

For many of my patients in Washington, D.C., that initial infection was a tick bite. Yet there are more than 300,000 new cases of Lyme disease a year across the country and only 10 to 20 percent of the people bitten become chronically ill. This means the vast majority – as many as 80 to 90 percent of those who have Lyme disease – get better.

The overwhelming number of kids who develop a strep infection will simply get better with antibiotics. Only a very small percentage develops PANDAS. Almost everyone has had mononucleosis, which can result in multiple sclerosis and ME/CFS, but only for a true minority of people. So, what is different about these people?

The answer is complicated and not yet fully understood. Like our psychological profile, our health itself is dependent on a combination of nature and nurture, or, as we doctors like to call it: genetics and environment.

Within our environment, a number of factors influence our health, including diet, toxins, and stress. The emotional and/or physical assaults a person endures and the way they survive them are also highly influential.

Each of these crucial elements builds up over time. They are reflected in what is known as the *allostatic load*, a measure of the stress and its impact on health. The evidence increasingly shows that high allostatic load has consequences for our health and well-being. It dramatically reduces our resilience, making us more susceptible to developing an autoimmune disease.[237]

LISTENING TO THE BODY

One of the techniques I use with patients is designed to help them reconnect with their bodies, while helping me understand the depth and extent of the trauma they are holding onto.

First, I ask them to rest comfortably on the table or in a chair while I take them through a quick relaxation technique, encouraging them to breathe deeply into their belly, while they imagine gathering their tension with each inhale and releasing it with every exhale. Then they relax each part of their body from their fingertips to their toes.

Since one of the essential requirements is that the person feels completely safe and in control, I assure them that they can stop the exercise any time they feel frightened or overwhelmed.

I then ask if there is any area of their body that needs attention. Typically, one area is experiencing discomfort. If several areas need attention, they choose one to start with.

The first time I took Janet through this exercise, she developed a severe stomach pain. When we started, she had pain and discomfort in many places, but no stomach pain. Shortly after we started, she was nauseous, close to vomiting, and almost doubled over with stomach pain.

I encouraged her to breathe into the pain, reminding her that she was safe. Soon the pain subsided, and she wanted to proceed. As she breathed into the area of pain, the discomfort got quite intense again, so we needed to allow time for her to breathe, feel safe, and not so overwhelmed.

At each stage, I asked, "What else is there?" The answer was a lot.

Shame, grief, guilt, and no small amount of anger – the list was long. It started with the realization of how unsafe and chaotic her house was when she younger. It extended into years of believing she was a failure and acting out in ways that were extremely self-destructive. It left her afraid to even think about a future. All of this did not come out in a single session but once the dam broke, we had a great deal of work to do aside from killing bugs and removing toxins.

I can do this work with my patients because I do not work alone. Our toolkit is a team of practitioners that include physicians with expertise in family medicine, pain medicine, functional medicine, physical therapists, an acupuncturist, a counselor skilled in individual and trauma therapy, a meditation instructor, and a nutritionist, in addition to coordinating care with outside specialists. People as sick as Janet require a village.

Obviously not everyone we see needs the attention of the whole team, but working as a team enables us to manage more complex patients. Working as a team has also helped all of us grow as healers. We learn a great deal from each other. The team also provides the opportunity to consult and support each other as we work through difficult clinical problems.

Often emotional wounds stored deep in the body emerge during this exercise that had not been apparent in the patients' histories. It takes time and trust to allow us to treat these wounds, since patients can be hiding them from both themselves and others. In the meantime, the body can be responding in very negative ways to these buried emotions. In this context, an attack on the self is not just a metaphor, it is clearly manifest in the immune system.

The power of this technique lets us engage with our patients in a very deep way, listening to our bodies and allowing us to more fully understand the dimensions of the illness.

I also use this technique for therapeutic guidance. In one patient who was unable to tolerate a number of medications, using this technique, we were able to understand what medication she could tolerate and even in what manner she could take the medication for it to work successfully.

Perhaps one of the most startling revelations came with a patient who got the message from her body, "It's the kidney, stupid!" She had struggled with chronic fatigue for several years and seen a number of physicians, yet all her testing had been normal. When this message came to her, we did an imaging of her kidney and found that a "silent" kidney stone had completely shut down her right kidney. After surgery to remove the stone, she improved immediately.

The body is a very complex place. While we are healthy, we strive for a quick fix whenever we get sick. Chronic illness is another beast. When it attacks unrelentingly and never leaves, it can be followed by a sense of betrayal and an attempt to escape from the body.

I get it. I have had the displeasure of kidney stones three times myself. Breathing deeply or easing into the pain only goes so far. Morphine was a godsend. But when the pain goes on, day after day, we need to connect with ourselves to find out everything we need to know about how exactly we are wounded and what we can do to heal. This is the most difficult thing I ask my chronically ill patients to do, though frankly it is the most important thing we do: sit and listen.

Please do not misunderstand; I am not saying that everyone with an autoimmune disease or a chronic disease is harboring deep-seated emotional traumas.

Chronic illness can be an immensely traumatic experience all by itself without any underlying emotional issues. It can slam on the brakes and put your life on hold. My patients have been forced to stop their education, stop their careers, and lose their independence. It often robs them of their sense of agency, power, and control. A world where disability has replaced ability is a very frightening place.

Healing requires attention to these experiences, as well as traumas lingering from the past. Connecting with our bodies allows us to do that part of the work.

Meditation is another way to listen. It offers us a place to abide quietly, free from the demands and distractions of the world around us. I recommend it for all my patients. For a long time, studies of mediation have shown it to have beneficial effects on health. Now we know that it also positively impacts our immune system.[238] When Janet introduced meditation to her daily routine, she reported that it gave her a greater sense of calm and control over her life.

So many people hold onto grudges that negatively affect their health that I have begun to introduce the concept of forgiveness into their healing regimens too. I am always impressed by how much I see their bodies relax, their pain decrease, and their mood become more optimistic once they made a decision to forgive themselves and others.

For Janet, getting in touch with her body through scans and meditation, along with the notion of releasing the past with forgiveness, had dramatic results. The feeling that her illness had imprisoned her began to dissipate. Moving beyond the negative assumptions she had nurtured in the past, she found the idea of a future had begun to take root.

As a result of all these efforts, while Janet has had to temporarily withdraw from school, she has already accomplished something she once believed would never be possible. She will miss a semester, but I am confident she will be back in the fall.

PART IV

A STEP-BY-STEP GUIDE TO RECOVERY

The first step toward getting somewhere is deciding you're not going to stay where you are.

~ JP Morgan

* * *

Now that you know about the nature of the problem, this Do-It-Yourself section will show you how to fix it. It is filled with the tests, supplements, and treatments that I have used for years to help my patients recover from autoimmune disease. For some tests and treatments, you will need to partner with doctors, but you will no longer need to approach doctors like a supplicant. The information provided in this chapter will make you an informed advocate for yourself and your own health.

Remember that with autoimmunity, each step in the process is essential. The infection, the things that set up your vulnerability to autoimmune disease, then the immune system itself must all be addressed. Unless they are each resolved, your autoimmune disease will flare back up again.

If you don't find and completely eliminate the infection, you will never restore your health, and autoimmunity will continue to keep you sick in one way or another. If you don't correct the sleep problems, gut imbalances, toxins, and traumas that made you vulnerable in the first place, you'll continue to be too unhealthy to regain your vitality. And if you don't carefully attend to your immune system to calm it back down after all the other issues have been cleared away, you will live in a precarious position – always prone to your body overreacting to the slightest challenge and stirring up these autoimmune issues all over again.

Whatever you do, don't skip a step. Do each one well, and recovery from autoimmunity is within your grasp.

CHAPTER 12

—

THE THREE STEPS

YOUR ROADMAP FOR RECOVERY

P art IV gives you the tools to help yourself, even when you
work hand-in-hand with your physician to coordinate
tests and treatments. Many times, you will be able to
identify and treat conditions by simply following the instructions I've given you here.

STEP ONE

Find and Eliminate the Infections

Because of the nature of the infections we are facing today,
testing is not always as straightforward as we would like. In
addition, it is not unusual for there to be several infections at
the same time. If you don't look, you will not find, and if you
look with the wrong test, you will not find. All testing has
limitations. That's why the labs and tests I describe in Part
IV are so important. With the right testing, follow-ups, and
treatment, you will be able to find, identify, and eliminate the
infections that triggered your autoimmune disease.

STEP TWO

Identify all the issues that made you sick or keep you sick

If you are suffering with an inflamed brain, the odds are that you have more than one of these issues setting you up. You must be diligent and search out all the problems, exterminate the pathogens, eliminate the toxins, repair your sleep, your gut, your mitochondria, and, most importantly, your immune system.

- Unhealthy sleep
- Gut imbalance
- Environmental toxins
- Emotional traumas

STEP THREE

Treat your over-reactive immune system

Once you have eliminated the infections and the issues that were making your brain and body vulnerable, the essential last step is to calm down your immune system.

This is the step that so many doctors miss. Autoimmunity indicates that your immune system has been over-reactive, so if you skip this step, the slightest thing can make it flare back up again.

Attend carefully to all three of these steps with the tests, treatments, supplements, and other recommendations in Part IV. With this vital information, your health and well-being are in your hands. Find a medical advocate in your area that you can trust and start this process together for the best results.

CHAPTER 13

—

ELIMINATE INFECTIONS

When patients come into my office suffering with chronic illness, the five most common undiagnosed infections I find are:

- Lyme disease
- Bartonella
- Babesia
- Epstein-Barr
- Mycoplasma infection

The key to these five infections is that they are not only missed but they can frequently also cause inappropriate activation of the acquired immune system, resulting in autoimmunity.

Testing and treatment for these five infections and the autoimmunity they can cause is controversial and complicated. There are unquestionably other infections that can be missed. I test for many others besides these five bugs depending on my patient's history and presentation.

My goal in this book is to arm you with enough knowledge to have a knowledgeable conversation with your physician.

Keep in mind that conditions like myalgic encephalomyelitis/ chronic fatigue syndrome, chronic pain, neuropsychiatric disorders, POTS, and PANS are the symptoms, not the disease.

LYME DISEASE

This disease is an infection transmitted by a tick that is infected with the bacterium Borrelia burgdorferi. Not all ticks carry this disease. The ticks that can infect you with Lyme disease are the blacklegged ticks also known as deer ticks.

Although the person bitten may never notice the tick or the bite itself, they soon begin to notice symptoms. Without treatment, the infection can spread to the heart, the joints and the nervous system.[239] An erosive arthritis somewhat like rheumatoid arthritis can take hold. At a later stage, it can become chronic progressive encephalitis or encephalomyelitis.[240]

Diagnosing Lyme disease is a challenge. Most people do not remember getting bitten by a tick. It's very small, about the size of the tip of a pencil (not the eraser). The classic "bull's eye rash," a round red rash with blank center only occurs 30 per cent of the time. Most people don't even remember it or mistake it for a fleeting allergic reaction.[241]

Testing for Lyme in most labs today is dependent on detection of antibodies (that is, the body's reaction to the bite). Antibodies don't develop in the blood for 2–3 weeks, so if the testing is performed too soon, the test may be normal while you are not. This is called a false negative because you have the disease, but the testing missed it. Other reasons for a false negative include:

- A suppressed immune system due to medications or Lyme disease itself.
- Antibiotics that partially eradicated Lyme disease, but not completely.
- Other tick-borne infections, such as anaplasmosis, Ehrlichiosis, Babesiosis, and Bartonellosis.

Traditionally, testing is done in two steps. The first step is to take a test called ELISA (Enzyme Linked Immunosorbent

Assay). This test was originally reported to be highly sensitive. If you had the disease, the test showed up positive almost all the time. But we now know that the ELISA test can be too insensitive and create a false negative result, telling us you don't have the disease when you do.

So, now a follow-up test is used to confirm the result of the ELISA test. The Western Blot tests for multiple antibodies to the disease. Too few antibodies or the wrong antibodies should confirm you are healthy, but there is an ongoing disagreement between experts as to which antibodies are important and how many constitute a positive Lyme test.

That is not the only problem. By combining the two tests, it was clear that the ELISA gives false positives about 50 percent of the time, as is later confirmed by the Western Blot. Physicians who don't know that tend to rely on the ELISA test and never confirm it with the Western Blot. So, they tell about half the people who have Lyme that they do not have the disease.[242]

If you think you have Lyme disease, talk to your physician. Request both the ELISA and the Western Blot to confirm its results. You may even explore a number of new testing strategies being developed.[243, 244] The FDA recently approved a new two-step test that eliminates the need for the Western Blot. Not all physicians are using it now, but you can always request it.

Additional testing for Lyme disease can be done at the following labs:

TEST: IgeneX - Borrelia (LYME) tests.
https://igenex.com/

TEST: Vibrant America - TickBorne 2.0 (Borrelia and co-infections).
https://www.vibrant-america.com/

If you have symptoms and you live in an area where Lyme is common, it's a good idea to get tested whether you remember being bitten by a tick or not. If you know you have been bitten, it's a good idea to get the test too, just in case. Be sure to wait for 2–3 weeks before you take it.

If you test positive and your doctor gives you antibiotics that solve the problem, count yourself fortunate. Most people (80 to 90 percent) never develop chronic Lyme disease.

Only 10 to 20 percent of people who become infected develop chronic Lyme disease, sometimes called Post-Treatment Lyme Disease Syndrome. It is much more severe and much harder to eradicate.

Although diagnostic testing and treatment are evolving, the controversy about Lyme among medical professionals is virulent enough that numerous articles have been written about "The Lyme Wars."[245] [246] Unfortunately, suffering patients are caught in the middle.

Treating Lyme is exceptionally complex. The Lyme bug itself exists in the body in three forms: spirochete, cystic, and persister. Each one requires a different set of antibiotics/medications. Often there are co-infections of Bartonella or Babesia that are exacerbating the problem but have not been identified. Because Lyme suppresses the immune system, old infections, such as Epstein-Barr, can reemerge and add a new layer of confusing symptoms on top of those created by Lyme. It is also not uncommon for environmental toxins, such as mold, to interfere with the body's ability to fight off the infection. In the struggle, the immune system can become overwhelmed and misfire, in which case, it is now part of the problem, and without addressing your damaged immune system, you will not heal.

I am a proud member of ILADS (International Lyme and Associated Disease Society, ILADS.org) and have been for many years. I believe that chronic Lyme is a real disease and that we now have some good treatment options to address the disease. Dr. Richard Horowitz has written two excellent books on tick-borne diseases and others are also available. I have also lectured on Lyme. In May 2019, The Foundation for Total Recovery co-sponsored a conference with Georgetown Medical School on autoimmune diseases of infectious etiology in which the tick-borne diseases were discussed at length.

ILADS defines chronic Lyme disease (CLD) as a multisystem illness with a wide range of symptoms and/or signs that are either continuously or intermittently present for a minimum of six months. The illness is the result of an active and ongoing infection by any of several pathogenic members of the Borrelia burgdorferi sensu lato complex. The infection has variable latency periods and signs, and symptoms may wax, wane, and migrate. CLD has two subcategories: CLD, untreated (CLD-U) and CLD, previously treated (CLD-PT). The latter requires that CLD manifestations persist or recur following treatment and are present continuously or in a relapsing/remitting pattern for a duration of six months or more.[247]

One tool that has been helpful in guiding our diagnosis of chronic Lyme is the Horowitz Multiple Systemic Infectious Disease Syndrome Questionnaire.[248] Taking the time to complete this questionnaire may provide you and your physician significant insight into your diagnosis, and with a proper diagnosis, get you on your road to recovery. This tool along with other lectures and more information on the diagnosis and treatment is available on our website.

In Chapter 5, you read about Bartonella, Babesia and other pathogens. Because most of my patients have been sick for years, it is not unusual for them to be infected with Lyme, Babesia, and Bartonella all at the same time.

BARTONELLA

There are multiple species of Bartonella and the testing for these bugs is far less than perfect, so I do several types of tests. As I've said earlier, the challenge is that these infections can hide inside the cells. They manipulate the immune system to avoid attack. They are known as persister bugs, which means they can hang around and cause the acquired immune system to go rogue, starting an autoimmune reaction.[249]

Bartonella behaves like a small animal that tears up your yard and hides every time you come out to find it. If it burrows underground, you may be able to find it with a sonar or infrared device. You may be able to track the trail of its scat (waste material) to its lair. But ultimately, each of these solutions is imperfect. Most likely, you will have to combine several approaches to find the critter. In the same way, you may need to combine the results of several different tests, the clues of your physical symptoms, and your response to treatment before you can find the Bartonella in your body and confirm the diagnosis.

Laboratory diagnosis alone can be tricky. Because this bug is so hard to find, I rely on two different labs that do multiple types of testing for this bug:

TEST: IgeneX - Bartonella tests.
https://igenex.com/
TEST: Galaxy Labs - Bartonella tests.
https://www.galaxydx.com/

BABESIA

This family of bugs is malaria-like protozoans. Babesia microti is most common. It invades and reproduces in the red blood cells. If you do not think about it, you won't look for it.

The symptoms from a viral illness can last from weeks to months. Some people have no symptoms at all. For others with compromised immune systems, it can be fatal.

The early infection can provoke intermittent fevers, fatigue, headaches, chills, muscle pain, nausea, vomiting, diarrhea, and depression. It doesn't help that a lot of other illnesses present the same way.[12] The most common complaints I hear are:

- Sweats (day or night)
- Chills
- Flushing
- Fever
- Cough
- Shortness of breath (air hunger)

Testing can be done again in the usual labs, but you need to do multiple types of testing. Again, I rely on:

TEST: IgeneX - The Co-Infection Panel.
https://igenex.com/

EPSTEIN-BARR VIRUS

Four antibodies can be tested when looking for Epstein-Barr. It causes mononucleosis, which is often called the "kissing disease" because it can be passed by intimate contact. Many of us caught the infection in high school. The fact is that almost everyone by the age of 25 has gotten the infection and has some antibodies to this virus.

TEST: Epstein-Barr antibodies

- **Viral capsid antigen-immunoglobin M** (VCA-IgM): If someone is positive for VCA-IgM antibodies, then it is likely that the person has an EBV infection, and it may be early in the course of the illness. These antibodies will go away in time.

- **Viral capsid antigen-IgG** (VCA-IgG): If this is positive, it means that an EBV infection has occurred recently or in the past. If the VCA-IgM is positive as well, then the infection is recent and ongoing. This antibody may be present for your entire life after an infection.
- **Epstein-Barr nuclear antigen** (EBNA): The presence of this antibody suggests a prior infection from EBV and typically lasts a lifetime.
- **Early Antigen-D** (EA-D, IgG): This is a very sensitive test for actively replicating viruses. While this antibody can be present in 10 to 30 percent of healthy people, it can also indicate a reactivation of an old EBV infection. If the VCA-IgM is negative and you are suffering with chronic fatigue syndrome, then this may be the cause of your ME/CFS.

TEST: Lab Tests Online
https://labtestsonline.org/tests/epstein-barr-virus-ebv-antibody-tests

MYCOPLASMA INFECTION

Mycoplasma is family of bacteria with over 200 species. Only 23 of them can cause disease, but three species are transmitted by ticks: mycoplasma pneumoniae, mycoplasma genitalium, and mycoplasma fermentans.

M. pneumoniae is the most common and the most well-known. A blood test is typically performed for mycoplasma infections, but the test can be inaccurate. If the symptoms persist, it is important to repeat testing periodically to find the bug.[20][21]

The common symptoms are respiratory: a cough, nasal congestion, and sore throat. It can also cause joint or muscle pain, as well as heart and neurologic symptoms.

TEST: Blood Test

Testing for a chronic mycoplasa infection can be complicated and controversial. As a screening test, I order a blood test for IgM and IgG antibodies. IgM, if positive, indicates either an active or recent infection, though the IgM can remain positive for upwards of a year after an acute infection. Elevated IgM can be found in patients with reactivated infections. While IgG is usually indicative of a past infection and may remain positive for years, exceptionally high results (this will be dependent on your lab) might suggest an ongoing chronic infection. If these tests are abnormal, you typically will repeat the test in 4–6 weeks to see if there is any change in the levels.

SUPPLEMENTS

Glutathione: The most abundant antioxidant in the brain is depleted in chronic illness. You can either take glutathione as a supplement or use N-acetyl cysteine, which helps the body make glutathione.

Epsom salt baths and infrared (IR) sauna: The magnesium in Epsom salt helps relax the muscles. Start with one pound in a bathtub of warm water and soak for 15 minutes. Sweating is one way we eliminate toxins. Both the baths and the IR sauna promote toxin elimination.

Massage for lymphatic drainage: Regular massage helps the body's immune system.

Vitamin D: Every cell in the body has a receptor for vitamin D. That makes vitamin D unique. It is involved in a wide range of activities in every part of the body. Vitamin D is necessary for a healthy immune system. We normally get it through the exposure of our skin to the sun. Vitamin D deficiency is widespread because we spend so much of our lives indoors and use sunscreens that indirectly block its production. It is a good idea to check your blood levels of vitamin D, maintaining a level of 50-80ng/ml is ideal.

Vitamin C: This vitamin is important to healthy immune function.[26] When taken orally, your digestive system will limit how much you can take. At higher dosages you will develop diarrhea. In my chronically ill patients, I recommend IV supplementation because the body can tolerate much higher dosages. (Be aware that some people have allergies to citrus from which most vitamin C is derived. Others have a genetic variant, glucose-6 phosphate dehydrogenase G6PD, which results in the lack of an enzyme that leads to damage to their red blood cells from high-dose vitamin C. A simple blood test can determine if you are missing this enzyme.)

Vitamin C in very high dosages given intravenously (7.5–50 gms) was shown in one study to be effective against chronic EBV infection.[30]

Magnesium: This mineral is essential for normal immune function and is frequently deficient. Magnesium levels in the blood are often normal, even when people are severely deficient. It is important to measure intracellular magnesium to determine deficiency. In chronically ill patients, I use IV magnesium therapy.

We all need 300–350 mg of magnesium a day. This amount is rarely present in our diets and, to make it worse, we are constantly depleting magnesium with alcohol, high-salt diets, exercise, stomach-acid inhibitors, and diuretics.

Several forms of oral magnesium irritate the digestive track. Magnesium L-threonate is readily absorbed, causes little stomach irritation, and has been shown to be helpful in chronic pain and brain function.[26][27]

Omega 3 Oils: I generally recommend 1,500 mg of a high-quality fish oil a day taken with food to influence inflammation and immunity.

Probiotics: Taking probiotics is essential whenever you are taking an antibiotic to help protect the functioning of the immune system and gut flora balance.

Selenium (Se): A trace element and **Vitamin E** are both important for normal functioning of the immune system. Deficiencies can both impair the body's ability to fight off a virus and actually make some viruses more dangerous.[31]

Cordyceps: It is a medicinal mushroom used in traditional Chinese medicine. It has been demonstrated to have a multitude of medical benefits, which include but are not limited to its use as an antimicrobial, antioxidant, and anti-cancer therapy.[31] Cordyceps has been demonstrated to have antiviral activity specifically against EBV.[33]

Antiviral medications: They have been reported to be useful in at least a subset of people suffering with ME/CFS associated with Epstein-Barr Virus (EBV). These medications include Valacyclovir and Valganciclovir.[34] [35]

We also use several supplements from Researched Nutritionals, including:

Transfer Factors Multi-Immune
Transfer Factor PlasMyc

Researched Nutritionals has developed a range of products that have unique actions to help our immune system perform optimally, and I have been pleased with both the quality of their products and their effectiveness for my patients.

https://www.researchednutritionals.com/

Although these infections are complex, my goal has not been to make you an expert in the field, but to help you be an informed partner on your road to healing from these complex illnesses. There is much you can and should do to help yourself to recover.

For a more extensive list of supplements for your immune system, feel free to check our website.

CHAPTER 14

—

HEAL YOUR IMMUNE SYSTEM

THE INNATE IMMUNE SYSTEM

In recent years, our understanding of the link between innate immunity and inflammation has become a vibrant new area of research. It impacts everything from gene regulation to chronic disease to cellular biology and physiology of the brain.[250] We have never been in a better position to apply our new insights about this connection. But there is little doubt that the most exciting breakthroughs are just over the horizon.

As you know, the adaptive immune system is invaluable to us. It represents the immunity we acquire through life. Any time there is inflammation in the body, the innate immune system is at work. When it becomes overstimulated, we need tools to calm it down. Otherwise, it can generate long-standing inflammatory issues that are far more difficult to quell.[251]

At this point, we have a limited ability to test the innate immune system itself, but two types of cells can give us insight into the level of inflammation being created in our bodies: mast cells and microglia.

MAST CELLS

Mast cells are part of the innate immune system and are scattered through our connective tissues, bone marrow, and blood vessels. We have known about them since German scientist Paul Ehrlich described them in 1878, but we did not understand their relationship to inflammation until the middle of the 20th century. Now we know that mast cells are key players in autoimmune diseases.[252]

Under stress, mast cells release substances called mediators that cause inflammation. When too many are released at the wrong time, it is called mast cell activation syndrome (MCAS).[253] Gradually, we are beginning to recognize that MCAS is a primary cause or component of many conditions, such as depression, anxiety, fibromyalgia, headaches, POTS, and Ehlers-Danlos syndrome (EDS).

TESTS
During an acute attack, perform these tests:
- Urine Test: N-Methylhistamine and PGD2
- Blood Serum Test: Tryptase

Please note that at the time of this writing, MCAS is diagnosed clinically, in person by a physician, more commonly than with a blood or urine test. With these characteristics, MCAS could be an underlying issue – or part of an underlying issue – for you.

Do your symptoms come and go? Do they vary in severity? Do you experience recurrent flushing, hives, asthma, cramping, diarrhea, headaches, brain fog, POTS, or rapid heartbeats? MCAS often affects two or more systems at a time, such as your lungs, your nervous system, your cardiovascular system, or your digestive system.

TREATMENT

With MCAS, each treatment must be tailored to the patient. Only a knowledgeable physician can find the right combination of supplements and medications to quiet the mast cell response.

SUPPLEMENTS

Palmitoylethanolamine (PEA) is a dietary supplement of a naturally occurring molecule found in egg yolks, soybeans, peanuts, and other foods. (https://store.kaplanclinic.com)

Neuroprotek is a supplement containing Luteolin, Quercetin and Rutin. (https://store.kaplanclinic.com)

MEDICATIONS

Multiple receptors for histamine (H1, 2, 3, 4) excite mast cells. Histamine 1 receptors require antihistamines. Histamine 2 receptors require stomach acid suppression.

Over-the-counter medications Claritin, Allegra, and Zyrtec are excellent H1 antihistamines. Pepcid AC and Tagamet are excellent H2 antihistamines, but they also block stomach acid as well. The H2 antihistamines can disrupt the gut microbiome, so you need to be careful.

Prescriptions such as Singulair or Cromolyn sodium can be useful, but I encourage you to partner with your physician in making these choices. You cannot do this part alone. My goal is to make you an educated partner in your own health care.

MICROGLIA

Microglia are very small cells in the brain that function primarily as immune cells. They are responsible for the activation of inflammation in the central nervous system. Neurological degenerative disorders, infectious diseases, and autoimmune diseases can be accompanied by the hyper-activation of these cells.[254]

PRESCRIPTIONS
Low dose naltrexone (0.5–4.5 mg a day)
Celebrex

ACTIVITIES
One of the best anti-inflammatory medicines for the brain is exercise. Meditation is a close second.

SUPPLEMENTS
There are in fact many supplements that have been found helpful for healing the microglia. Some of the best we have found are listed below.

- Resveratrol
- Curcumin
- Ginseng
- Green tea
- Melatonin
- Vitamin D
- Palmitoylethanolamine (PEA)

THE ACQUIRED IMMUNE SYSTEM
The first question to ask is if your acquired immune system is activated and working well. The acquired immune system is a great, big system, and we are still trying to understand exactly how to test for dysfunction and how to respond to the testing we get. This is why we see a diagnosis such as seronegative rheumatoid arthritis. What this means is that you have all the symptoms and some of the tests (such as x-rays) that would be consistent with rheumatoid arthritis, but when we test your immune system, the usual testing that should be abnormal to make the diagnosis of rheumatoid arthritis, is normal. Go figure.

TESTS

Immunoglobins (Ig)

These antibodies fight bacteria, viruses, and other invaders. Having too many or too few causes a problem. You need just the right balance.

The major classes of immunoglobins are Total IgG, IgA, IgM, IgE (G.A.M.E.). When different classes are elevated, they result in different effects. Elevated IgE, for instance, most commonly indicates allergies but are also seen in other conditions such as parasitic infections. The Immunoglobin G class is divided into subfractions 1, 2, 3, 4.

If the test reveals abnormal levels of any classes or subclasses of immunoglobin, it suggests that your immune system is not up to par. In that case, seek out further testing with an immunologist.

Antinuclear antibody (ANA)

This test measures antinuclear antibodies (ANA) in titers (such as 1:32). The higher the titer, the more ANA in the blood and the more likely you have an autoimmune disease.

High ANA is associated with systemic lupus erythematosus (SLE), a type of autoimmune disease, but not definitive. Low titers annoy us to no end because in isolation – meaning, without other physical or laboratory findings – it is not clear whether they are important or not. For instance, a viral infection may cause a temporary elevation of the ANA.

To help put this test in perspective, it may be helpful to test inflammatory markers such as the sedimentation rate (sed rate) and C-reactive proteins (CRP). Working with your physician, you can understand the various interpretations in relation to your own condition.

AUTOIMMUNITY TRIGGERED BY INFECTION

TEST: The Cunningham Panel

A classic blood test, The Cunningham Panel, measures the levels of autoantibodies circulating in the blood. When levels are elevated, it can indicate infection-driven autoimmunity.[255] It was developed by Dr. Madeleine Cunningham at the University of Oklahoma.

When unusual psychiatric symptoms appear, The Cunningham Panel can be used to determine whether the origin is physical or psychological.

Infections like the flu, strep, pneumonia, or even sinusitis can trigger autoimmunity and brain inflammation in vulnerable people. When this occurs, neurological and psychological symptoms can flare up. These often mimic depression, obsessive compulsive disorder, ADHD, autism spectrum disorder, and other autoimmune conditions.[256]

Dr. Kiki Chang, Professor of Psychiatry and Behavioral Sciences at Stanford University Medical School, says, "We can't say how many kids with psychiatric symptoms have a behavioral, immune, or inflammatory component to their disorder, but given the burgeoning research indicating that inflammation drives mood disorders and other psychiatric problems, it's likely to be a large subset of children and even adults diagnosed with psychiatric illnesses."[257] The presence of these antibodies has been correlated with pediatric autoimmune neuropsychiatric disorder (known as PANDAS when it is caused by a streptococcal infection and PANS when caused by other infections).

While there has been some controversy about the validity of The Cunningham Panel, I had the privilege of being one of the coauthors on a paper published in the *Journal of Immunology* validating its clinical importance and usefulness.[258]

Currently, The Cunningham Panel is only approved for children. A number of physicians around the country, myself included, have found that the panel is also valid in diagnosing adults who are suffering with autoimmune brain disorders resulting from infection. We are working toward formal approval of this panel for adults. But in the meantime, I and many others find this test invaluable in diagnosing and guiding the treatments of adults as well as children.

The panel is available through Moleculera Labs in Oklahoma. This lab has pioneered advanced testing services to help identify the causes of autoimmune dysfunction. In many cases, obsessive compulsive disorder (OCD), tics, anxiety, attention deficit hyperactivity disorder (ADHD), and autism spectrum disorder (ASD) prove to be caused by treatable autoimmune conditions, triggered by everyday infections.[259]

Moleculara Labs https://www.moleculeralabs.com/cunningham-panel-pandas-pans-testing/

TEST: CellTrend Antibodies

While The Cunningham Panel tests for antibodies that target the brain, CellTrend Antibodies target the peripheral nerves outside the brain. This antibody test was designed by a German company called CellTrend.

It is now clear from the research, but not widely appreciated in the medical profession, that a large subset, possibly the majority of patients with fibromyalgia, complex regional pain syndrome (CRPS), and postural orthostatic hypotension (POTS), are suffering with an autoimmune disease that attacks the peripheral nerves (those nerves that are outside of the brain and the spinal cord). Failure to identify those who have been diagnosed with these conditions who are suffering with a dysfunction of their acquired immune system results in failure to treat properly. CellTrend antibody panels are the best tests available for identifying the antibodies found in the subset of patients with conditions such as fibromyalgia, CRPS, and POTS, who have an autoimmune disorder attacking the nerves outside of the brain.

Autoimmunity is complicated. Many physicians do not understand the nature of the problem and do not have the tools to make the diagnosis. As a result, too many people are suffering because of our ignorance. Tests like these will help you begin to find a solution.

CellTrend https://www.celltrend.de/en/

TEST FOR POTS

You can diagnose POTS in two ways. One is high-tech, the other is old-school.

If you prefer high-tech, see a cardiologist to get a tilt-table test. The tilt-table test involves lying secured to a flat table which is then moved from a flat position to an almost upright position. Your blood pressure and pulse will be measured during this process. If you'd rather go old-school, get a blood pressure wrist cuff at your local drug store. Simply lie flat without moving for five minutes, then check your pulse and blood pressure. Next stand up and without moving around, check it again three minutes later, then five minutes later, then ten minutes later. To be on the safe side, make sure someone is with you should you feel faint. If your blood pressure remains stable but your heart rate increases by more than 30 beats for adults or 40 beats for teenagers when you go from lying down to standing, you most likely have POTS. If your standing heart rate is 120 beats a minute within ten minutes, you may have POTS. If your blood pressure significantly drops during this test, you have another problem. All of these issues require medical attention but are different diagnoses and treated differently.[260]

TREAMENTS

Many of these treatments, like the diagnoses themselves, are fraught with complexity and controversy. Because brain inflammation is caused by the reaction of the acquired immune system to an infection, the most important thing you must do is eradicate the infection. At the same time, you also need to soothe the overactive immune response. The therapies below are directed at the immune system specifically.

MEDICATIONS

Metformin: Nearly 120 million people worldwide are taking metformin.[261] It is most commonly used to treat prediabetes or Type 2 diabetes. Recently, it has been touted by the anti-aging community to slow the aging process. It is useful in treating autoimmunity because metformin helps modulate an overactive acquired immune system.[262] Hot off the presses as of this writing is a study that suggests that metformin may mitigate the severity of Covid-19. Diabetics who developed Covid-19 and were being treated with metformin had dramatically milder cases.[263] Pay attention to this drug. I expect it will find an increasingly wide range of uses in the future.

Intravenous Immunoglobulin (IV-IG)

Intravenous immunoglobulin (IV-IG) is an intravenous solution consisting of highly purified, polyclonal IgG antibodies from the plasma of tens of thousands of donors.[264]

This treatment boosts immunity to fight infection for those who are immunocompromised. With additional antibodies, the body is better able to fight infection.

Remarkably effective, it can raise low red blood cell counts in those with autoimmunity, prevent the white blood cells from destroying the red blood cells in those with lupus, and block the destruction of muscle cells by the immune system in those with myositis.[265]

That said, it is not a benign treatment, and it is very expensive. Insurance companies approve this treatment for only a few conditions, such as chronic inflammatory demyelinating polyneuropathy (CIDP). CIDP is an autoimmune disease that targets the peripheral nerves and can be set off by Lyme disease. It causes loss of sensation and weakness in peripheral nerves. Occasionally, insurance companies will approve the treatment for PANS and PANDAS as well.

At The Kaplan Center, we have found it very helpful for many of our patients with autoimmune diseases caused by infections that affect the nervous system.

Plasmapheresis

Pheresis is a process that involves "washing" the blood of antibodies. Blood is drawn, filtered, and returned to the body. In that process, the plasma, platelets, red blood cells, and/or white blood cells may be separated. This plasma exchange literally removes harmful substances from the blood. In autoimmune disorders, it can even help discourage the body from producing harmful antibodies.[266]

The entire process takes two to three hours and may need to be repeated periodically. It is done at a hospital by physicians specially trained in the procedure. We send our more complicated PANDAS and PANS patients for this procedure with good results.

Rituximab

Known by the brand names Rituxan, Ruxience, or Truxima, this chemotherapy medication shuts down a part of the acquired immune system.

It is the most widely used drug for lymphoma but is also approved for rheumatoid arthritis. Many physicians use it off-label to treat autoimmune diseases, such as multiple sclerosis,[267] systemic lupus erythematosus, chronic inflammatory demyelinating polyneuropathy, and autoimmune anemia.[268]

It is controversial, expensive, and can have severe side effects, so use caution when considering it. Despite all that, it has been a lifesaver for many patients suffering with PANS, PANDAS, demyelinating polyneuropathy, and ME/CFS.[269]

REGENERATIVE THERAPIES
Stem Cells
Stem cells are the origin of all the tissue in our bodies. Because of their great creative ability, they have been shown to help your body repair itself. Stem cells have been used to repair both heart tissue damaged by heart attacks and brain tissue damaged by strokes. At The Kaplan Center, we have used stem cells to help repair joints in patients with arthritis.

Stem cells can be harvested from bone marrow or fatty tissue called autologous ("from ourselves") cells. They can also be taken from umbilical cord blood called allograft ("tissue from another").

While it was initially suspected that stem cells would work by simply replacing the cells that were damaged, it now appears that they incite a growth reaction that repairs damaged tissue.[270] In animals, stem cell therapy has already induced powerful healing in autoimmune disorders.[271]

We are only beginning to discover how we can work together with stem cells to create remarkable healing. We know that they modulate the immune system by reducing its pathological responses and retaining its ability to fight disease. Instead of suppressing the entire immune response, they act as local mediators. They also promote the production of immune cells that protect the body from attacking itself.[272]

Stem cells show great promise in treating autoimmune diseases. How they may work is still being debated, but it appears that they can get the immune system to stop producing antibodies that are attacking our own tissue while having an anti-inflammatory and reparative effect on tissues that have been damaged. A remarkable feat![273]

Exosomes

The rapidly advancing profusion of evidence now suggests that exosomes play an important role in autoimmune diseases. Only a few decades ago, they were thought to stimulate immune response. Physicians who wondered if they could be used as biomarkers or therapeutic agents for autoimmune disorders were on the right track.[274]

What we do know is that exosomes are small vesicles secreted by the cells in bodily fluids. They are clearly involved in inflammation, immune signaling, and angiogenesis. Many physicians consider them to be a promising new tool for the delivery of therapies, thanks to their stability, biocompatibility, and stealth capacity.

Think of an exosome as a way to cut out the stem cell middleman and get to the good stuff – in really tiny packets. The "good stuff" – anti-inflammatory, growth, and repair factors – is just as possible for exosomes as stem cells.

The advantage is that exosomes are plentiful. Since they do not have a cell wall as stem cells do, they should, theoretically, be much safer than stem cells.

According to the U.S. Food and Drug Administration, stem cell therapies do have the potential "to repair, restore, replace, and regenerate cells, and could possibly be used to treat many medical conditions and diseases." The primary danger arises from unscrupulous stem cell clinics. When the therapies are FDA-approved, they appear to be very safe.[275]

Research on both stem cell and exosomes therapies is still preliminary, but it is an exploding field full of promise. This is truly a new and very exciting frontier.

—

CHAPTER 15

HEAL YOUR SLEEP

First, we need to make sure you are getting proper sleep. To optimize your sleep, you need to regularly go to bed at the same time every night. Our bodies are creatures of habit. Whether or not we're consciously aware of it, they are operating in harmony with the rotation of the Earth to create a natural, circadian rhythm that coordinates our sleep-wake cycle with the movement of the planet every 24 hours.

Don't mess with that. The more chaotic your bedtime is, the worse the quality of your sleep will be. Whatever your personal inclinations or the demands of your schedule or your kids, the fact is that our bodies are meant to sync with the Earth's rotation. Work with that and you will reap the benefits of a good night's sleep of seven to nine hours.

If you have trouble falling asleep, staying asleep, waking too early, or waking in the night, try these adjustments to aid your sleep.

- **Daily Exercise.** Regular exercise creates a healthier body that naturally falls asleep more easily. Each person is different, but for most, it's a good idea to avoid exercise within four hours of going to bed.

- **Limit Caffeine.** One of the surest ways to know that you are drinking too much caffeine for your body is when you have trouble falling asleep or you get the feeling that you're sleeping lightly. Studies show that caffeine can delay your body's sleep clock and reduce the amount of deep sleep you achieve at night.[276]

- **Blue Light.** Turn off all electronics an hour before bedtime.
- **Room temperature.** Ideally, your night temperature should be between 60–68 degrees Fahrenheit.
- **Sleep Sounds.** Apps like Calm, Rain, Slumber, Fall Asleep, Insomnia are designed to produce soothing sounds to help you fall asleep.

My patients who suffer from fatigue often ask me whether naps are a good idea. It depends on the person. Short power naps of 30 minutes to 90 minutes (which is roughly a full sleep cycle) can be beneficial, especially if you have not gotten enough rest the night before.

Try not to nap after 3:00 PM. Longer naps tend to leave you feeling groggy or interfere with your sleep at night. If you have ME/CFS, think of these guidelines as goals and do the best you can. The goal is to maximize your brain's ability to detox and minimize inflammation.

TESTING

Two free tests are available on my site at www.kaplanclinic.com

- The Epworth Sleepiness Scale
- The Pittsburgh Sleep Quality Index (PSQI)

The Epworth is a quick questionnaire to screen for sleep apnea. If you score over ten on this test, there is a good chance you have sleep apnea and need to talk with your physician about more advanced testing. The PSQI is a short questionnaire that provides an excellent, overall objective test to evaluate the quality of your sleep.

Any of a number of devices can track your quality of sleep. Most are watches. But frankly, the best of the bunch is a ring called the OURA (https://ouraring.com).

SUPPLEMENTS

My best recommendations for sleep supplements are these:

- **Melatonin:** 0.1-10 mg at bedtime.
- **Magnesium taurate:** Magnesium comes in several forms. Magnesium taurate is best for sleep issues. It is less prone to cause diarrhea and has the best brain absorption.[277]
- **Valerian root:** 300–600 mg one to two hours prior to bedtime.
- **5-Hydroxytryptophane (5HTP):** 100–300mg at bedtime.
- **Glycine:** 3gm one hour before bedtime.
- **L-Theanine:** 200–400 mg morning and evening.

These doses are for adults only. Supplements can interact with medications you may be taking, or you may be allergic or have a sensitivity the supplement or additive, so check with your physician before starting anything new. Side effects, while unusual, such as headaches, stomach upset, and other issues, are possible.

MEDICATION

Your physician will be able to recommend the appropriate medication to help you sleep. What I like about the medications below is that they tend to preserve the sleep cycle, are non-addictive, and can frequently alleviate pain as well. This is by no means a complete list of all available medications that help with sleep.

Too frequently, physicians think sleep problem means a prescription of a sleep medication. There is not a lot of thought about the physiology of sleep. Ideally, your physician will begin by taking a good history of your sleep issues to understand your distinctive situation and tailor your treatment accordingly.

These medications are not the most common medications for sleep, and they should only be taken under the supervision of a physician.

- Nortriptyline (Pamelor) or Amitriptyline
- Doxepin (Sinequan) low-dose
- Gabapentin (Neurontin)
- Low-dose Naltrexone
- Trazodone (Desyrel)

INSOMNIA TREATMENT

Relaxation Techniques

Breathing exercises, guided imagery, and meditation techniques can help you relax before going to sleep. Progressive muscle relaxation techniques used to alternatively relax, tense, and relax your muscles can be very effective in inducing sleep and deep relaxation.

Stimulus Patterns

You can train your mind to associate the time of day, the nighttime routine, and the bedroom with sleep. Some stimulus trainers recommend getting up if you are awake for more than 20 minutes, so you do not develop the habit of lying awake in bed. Going to sleep at the same time every night and getting up at the same time reinforces the pattern.

Cognitive Behavioral Therapy (CBT)

The Mayo Clinic recommends cognitive behavioral therapy as

the psychotherapy of choice for insomnia. A simple technique that requires limited sessions to achieve results, it has proven to be effective with chronic sleep issues.[278]

A CBT therapist will provide you with a structured program for identifying any thoughts that are making your sleep problems worse and will help you replace them with thoughts and behaviors that promote good sleep. If thoughts or behaviors are at the root of your poor sleep, CBT has the benefit of resolving the problem by eliminating the underlying cause.[279]

Biofeedback
There are several biofeedback devices that can help you fall asleep faster and stay asleep. These devices measure your brain waves, and use visual and auditory feedback to help restore your sleep to a normal night's sleep without medication. Most of these devices help with relaxation in general.

URGOnight (https://www.urgonight.com)
This device is designed to help improve sleep. With regular use three times a week for 20 minutes over several weeks, it will help you get to sleep faster and stay asleep.

Light Therapy
One of the most helpful solutions for jet lag is light therapy. One of our favorites for resetting and improving your sleep-wake cycle is: **Pegasi glasses** (https://www.pegasiglasses.com)

Blue Light Glasses
LEDs from our computers and devices emit a blue light, which interferes with our production of melatonin and inhibits our ability to fall asleep.[280] By wearing glasses that block blue light emissions in the evenings, this effect can be avoided.

Acupuncture

Consider acupuncture if you are having trouble sleeping. It has been shown to be of help in a number of studies. [281, 282]

Meditation

The research is strong that regular meditation can improve your sleep. [283]

SLEEP APNEA TREATMENT

CPAP Machine

For years, this machine has been the gold standard for sleep apnea treatment. CPAP (continuous positive airway pressure), BiPAP (bilevel positive airway pressure), VPAP (variable positive airway pressure), and others are available, but they all serve the same purpose. Each one is appropriate for a different type of sleep apnea, so it is important to have a clear diagnosis and get the machine that will be most helpful to you.

Daytime sleepiness, heart function, hypertension, and quality of life improve dramatically with this treatment. Sleep apnea is greatly reduced, which results in restful sleep and significantly decreases the chances of more serious health problems. [284]

A wide variety of breathing masks are available for moderate to severe sleep apnea. The most common masks are worn snugly over the nose. The air pressure creates a mild suction in your mouth, which tends to keep your mouth closed, but those who still manage to breathe through their mouth can use a mask that covers both the nose and the mouth.

The CPAP machine sends pressurized air flowing through a hose continuously or intermittently into your nose. This pressure prevents your airway from collapsing and interrupting your breathing as you sleep.

Sleep apnea sufferers who stop using the CPAP expose themselves to a serious risk of developing other health problems, such as high blood pressure, heart attack, stroke, and diabetes. Yet despite these consequences, many people stop using it. In one long-term study, half of the patients given a CPAP machine were not using it. Most had never even filled the prescription! The other half used it and derived benefits from it. At least 25 percent of all patients discontinue CPAP therapy. Combined with those who were prescribed the device, but never used it, the long-term compliance rate is only 54 percent.[285]

Yet the device can literally make the difference between a long life and one cut short by health problems and poor sleep. The elimination of sleep apnea can have a profoundly energizing effect on your life and health. It is remarkable the difference it makes when you have enough sleep – not to mention getting oxygen to your brain and other organs every night.

Oral Appliances

To date, there are more than 100 different FDA-approved oral appliances for obstructive sleep apnea. They are worn in the mouth, like a sports or night guard. The appliance keeps the lower jaw forward slightly to hold the airway open, while preventing your tongue from relaxing enough to block your throat and the muscles in your upper airway from collapsing to block your airway.[286]

These appliances are often called sleep apnea mouth guards, jaw advancing devices (JAD), or mandibular advancement devices (MAD). They are custom-made by dentists.

Unfortunately, if you have an issue with hypermobile joints or TMJD (temporal mandibular joint disorder), this device is not a good choice for you.

TMJD CHECKLIST

- Does your jaw click or pop?
- Does your jaw ever lock?
- Do you have jaw or ear pain when chewing?
- Do awaken with a headache in the morning?
- Do you get ringing in your ears?
- Do you feel dizzy or lightheaded on a regular basis?
- Are you limited on how wide you can open your jaw? (A normal jaw opening should allow you to insert three fingers between your upper and lower front teeth.)
- If you answered yes to any of these questions, you need to check with your dentist about the possibility that you have TMJD. If you have headaches or facial pain, checking for TMJD should always be considered.

NARCOLEPSY TREATMENT

One of my patients, Fiona, was diagnosed with narcolepsy by a sleep specialist, who put her on a myriad of amphetamines for more than three years. The sleep specialist's theory was that increasing her alertness during the day would make her sleepier at night. No attempt was ever made to understand, much less cure, her inability to achieve REM sleep at night.

On her first visit to my office, I prescribed Xyrem, a drug that helps regulate sleep. Soon we were able to wean her off the addictive amphetamines that kept her alert all day but that did not address the underlying disease issue.

"Prior to taking Xyrem," Fiona said, "I would fall asleep anywhere anytime and sleep for very long periods without ever feeling rested. I could easily sleep 18–20 hours at a stretch. I would still wake up feeling exhausted." It was no way to live, and it kept her brain in an inflamed, agitated state. Today, after six years on Xyrem, Fiona marvels at the dramatic impact it's had on her life. "I am still often tired, but I don't fall asleep during conversations, at traffic lights, during sex, or at family gatherings – all of which used to be common occurrences!"

Ultimately, the treatment is medical. While we cannot cure narcolepsy, we can control it. Modafinil is typically the first medication prescribed. It is a stimulant with fewer side effects and addictive properties than the older amphetamine-like medications. There are now three medications that specifically treat narcolepsy. It is not infrequent that combinations of medications are needed to get the best results. The medication I prefer is sodium oxybate (Xyrem).

Its availability is restricted because it is somewhat similar to gamma-hydroxybutyric acid (also known as the "date rape drug") and since it is only approved for narcolepsy with cataplexy and/or daytime hypersomnolence, insurance companies will not cover the drug for other diagnoses. But it is still the best drug available for restoring sleep in Stages 3 and 4 (slow wave). Remember, as we said above, Stages 3 and 4 are the most important stages for helping the brain detoxify. The most important thing is that if you suspect you have narcolepsy, speak to your physician to get properly diagnosed and treated.

CHAPTER 16

—

HEAL YOUR GUT

There are three essential things to keep in mind about how critical the health of our gut is to the health of our immune system and brain.

First, approximately 70 percent of our immune system is located in the cells lining the wall of our gut. Thus, an unhealthy gut equals an unhealthy immune system.

Second, remember that there is a fairly direct relationship between the health of the gut wall (the gut-blood barrier) and the barrier that separates and protects the brain from bad things in our blood stream (blood-brain barrier). Thus, an unhealthy gut-blood barrier equals an unhealthy blood-brain barrier.

Third, there is a great deal of information that moves from the gut to the brain through a variety of channels, and each organ helps regulate the other. Thus, an unhealthy gut equals an unhealthy brain.[287, 288]

Step 1: FOOD ISSUES

There are three issues here. First, there are foods that you are truly allergic to. This type of allergy is mediated by an immunoglobin called IgE. These reactions vary from nasal congestion to hives to anaphylaxis. The onset is fairly immediate. Think about allergies to peanuts and shellfish. To identify these foods, you need to work with a physician who does food allergy testing.

CELIAC DISEASE

Celiac disease is an autoimmune disease that causes a reaction to foods containing gluten. It is most likely caused by a viral infection in a genetically predisposed person.[289]

We used to think that celiac disease showed up exclusively in children. The most common age of diagnosis is now between 40 and 60 years old. Celiac disease is estimated to impact over one million people in the United States. Studies suggest that over 95 percent of people who have celiac disease have not been diagnosed.[290]

I test people for celiac disease on a fairly regular basis in my practice. Typically, people with celiac disease have lots of intestinal problems like bloating, gas, and diarrhea, but sometimes the only symptom is depression or otherwise unexplained damage of the peripheral nerves. As I explained earlier in the book, I have "cured" depression by treating a young man with previously undiagnosed celiac disease.

TEST: Tissue Transglutaminase IgA Antibody
Test for anti-tTG-IgA and total IgA. If you are IgA-deficient, you may get a false negative.

TEST: Endomysial antibodies (EMA)
If this test is positive, there is a high probability that you have celiac disease. More definitive testing can be obtained by doing an endoscopic examination of the intestine.

TEST: Elimination Diet

Another method of testing is to completely eliminate all sources of gluten from your diet for a month and see how you feel. You may feel better regardless, since many people are gluten-intolerant without having celiac disease. If that's the case, I would recommend staying off gluten in general.

If you check the antibodies again after three months of a gluten-free diet and the levels are normal, you most likely have celiac disease, and it is imperative that you avoid gluten in all forms.

If you have celiac disease, you have an autoimmune disease that is triggered by eating gluten. This is very different than having gluten intolerance. The difference? Simply put, celiac disease may kill you, while gluten intolerance will annoy you. Still a problem, but on a very different scale. Celiac disease can also cause leaky gut, which we will get to in a minute.

Testing for celiac disease is accomplished by blood test and/ or biopsy of the small intestine by a gastroenterologist. The blood tests for celiac disease are available through any commercial lab but require a physician's order.

Some people have cross reactivity to other foods as a result of the damage to the small intestines from celiac disease. It is equally important to eliminate these foods to stop the ongoing inflammation in your intestines. The labs we use to test for cross-reactive foods are Vibrant America and Cyrex Labs which is a Clinical Immunology Laboratory specializing in functional immunology and autoimmunity.

Vibrant America: (https://www.vibrant-america.com/)
Cyrex Labs: (https://www.cyrexlabs.com/)

Treatment is to eliminate any and all sources of gluten and reactive foods found on testing. You also need to be under the care of a physician who understands celiac disease.

Fructose Malabsorption

Fructose is a sugar that is naturally found in fruits, some vegetables, and honey. It is also used as a sweetener in some beverages. Fructose malabsorption is when your gut is unable to break down the fructose during digestion. The result is gas, bloating, abdominal pain, and diarrhea.

Fructose intolerance can be caused by a rare inherited disorder but is more commonly acquired because of excess intake of alcohol, caffeine, high intake of refined/processed foods, a gastrointestinal infection and stress.[291] Fructose intolerance can thus be caused by, and is also a cause of, leaky gut.

Diagnosis of fructose malabsorption is typically by a breath test that measures the production of hydrogen and methane after eating a high fructose meal. This should be performed under the direction of your physician or a licensed nutritionist.

Aerodiagnostics: (https://aerodiagnostics.com/#service)

Treatment is primarily a low FODMAP diet. FODMAP stands for Fermentable Oligosaccharides, Disaccharides, Monosaccharides, and Polyols. It is a very effective diet for reducing inflammation, but it is best to work with a nutritionist for a diet tailored to your body.

https://www.healthline.com/nutrition/low-fodmap-diet

Acquired Food Allergies or Sensitivities

If your gut is inflamed, it will be leaky. As I explained earlier, a leaky gut is when the cells that make up the lining of the gut start to swell and separate opening spaces that should be "tight" and allowing large, incompletely digested molecules of food to pass into the blood stream. Your immune system looks at these large partially digested molecules and assumes they are invaders and makes antibodies to them. The result is reactions to foods you would not normally be allergic to if the lining of your gut were healthy.

Almost all of my patients suffer with a leaky gut as a result of their illness and the multiple treatments they have been subjected to in their search for a solution. Continuing to eat foods to which you have become sensitized will keep your gut, your immune system, and all of you inflamed. To heal your immune system and your brain, you will need to heal your gut. Once the gut is healed, many of the foods you identify as being sensitive to will stop being a problem after several months, and you will be able to enjoy a more varied diet again.

The elimination diet helps you identify foods to which your immune system has become hyper-sensitized. It is the easiest and most basic way to uncover adverse food reactions that may be contributing to various conditions such as digestive issues, depression, mood swings, eczema, skin irritation, asthma, headaches, chronic sinus drainage, low energy, joint aches, and weight gain.

Food reactions are frequently underestimated when we are trying to manage and treat a chronic condition, and we don't generally realize how awful we were feeling until we remove the food trigger. Why is that? Generally speaking, we are more diligent if some reactions happen immediately after eating a food, causing an allergy. However, we rarely associate our joint pain to eating a particular food, because symptoms may be delayed by several hours or even days.

So how do we do an elimination diet? Okay, all you need is three to four weeks of dedication and compliance to remove the major food allergens completely, then re-challenge those foods, and, most importantly, keep a food/symptom tracker to write down all the reactions. Let's go back to the foods that we need to eliminate: gluten, dairy, eggs, shellfish, peanuts, tree nuts, corn, and soy.

In addition to the major food allergens, I suggest to patients that they also eliminate caffeine, chocolate, and alcohol.

I'm sure you're wondering now about what you CAN eat. Well, plenty of vegetables, fruits, olive oil, or ghee for the fat, non-dairy substitutes such as almond, coconut, and any other nut milk/cheese. Also, all other protein sources such as lamb, wild game, fish, and poultry.

The reintroduction phase is simply adding back one food at a time from the eliminated list, choose the one food that you missed the most to reintroduce first. Eat that food abundantly for one day, while continuing with the elimination of the other foods.

Notice any symptoms that may appear for the next 48 hours, not only digestive symptoms, but any joint and muscle pain, sleepiness, headaches, etc.

Now, if the food you reintroduced caused worsening of your symptoms, you can conclude that it is a trigger and needs to be avoided for at least three months. If no symptoms are noticed, it means that it is a safe food, and you can keep it in your diet. After that, you can continue reintroducing one food after the other in the same manner and writing down any symptoms you experience. At the end you will have a better idea about which foods affect you, and you will be able to limit or eliminate them.

TEST: Allergies or Sensitivities

There are two types of food allergy tests, which evaluate which portion of the immune system is being activated. Type 1 food allergy tests for Immunoglobin E production. This is the classic allergy where if you eat a food you are allergic to, you develop a fairly immediate reaction in seconds to minutes, and where you can develop a variety of symptoms ranging from swelling, hives, or even anaphylactic shock. I used to love eggplant, but am now allergic, developing scratchy throat, brain fog, and nasal congestion. The response is quick, and the association is clear. An allergist may perform this test to confirm the specific food to which you are allergic.

The second type of allergy is caused by activation of Immunoglobin G (IgG) and produces symptoms that may not show up until up to three days after you have eaten the food. Foods that cause a delayed reaction can cause you to be in a chronic inflammatory state with issues such as headaches, irritable bowel symptoms, and chronic fatigue, and can cause you to gain weight. If you start an elimination diet and quickly lose five or more pounds the first few days, it is because you were eating foods that you are allergic to, and which cause swelling. Eliminating the food allows you to eliminate the water you were retaining because of the allergic reaction.

TEST: Genetic Gut Microbiome
Viome (https://www.viome.com)
A new type of testing that I believe will revolutionize our ability to customize a diet that is ideal for you as well as helping us to identify some of your health risks is looking at the genetics of your gut microbiome. We are all individuals, and one person's ideal diet may be poison for another. Viome is the first company that analyzes the genetics and epigenetics of the gut microbiome. What this means is that they can actually make dietary recommendations specific to how your microbiome digests your food.

We are on the verge of a revolution driven by all kinds of genetic testing, and this company is the first in this field of analyzing our gut microbiome. This is also one of those companies that is working with machine learning. What this means is that the more people they test, the better the testing gets because it "learns" as it gets more data. What this testing is able to tell us about our gut health and ideal diets today is only the beginning of what it will be able to tell us in the years to come. The data looks pretty good to me now to be of use.

I know that given my genetics, I am at risk for gout and, by experience, kidney stones. This test actually identified both these risks and was also able to outline a specific diet to help me from ever developing gout and preventing further kidney stones. It's not an especially expensive test, and I believe it will revolutionize our ability to truly institute individualized medicine. This test can be ordered by you directly from the company but we recommend reviewing the results with a qualified nutritionist or other health professional.

Step 2. GUT PATHOGENS

If you have worms or other parasites in your gut, these infections need to be eliminated. The conventional testing looking for these critters is poor and frequently misses the parasite. One of my patients became crippled by a roundworm infection called Strongyloidiasis that was missed in the initial testing. There are two labs that I use for parasite testing; both require stool samples, and I will frequently have patients do both because these critters can be difficult to find.

Genova Diagnostics GI Effects comprehensive test
https://www.gdx.net/
Parasitology Center Inc.
https://www.parasitetesting.com

TREATMENT
There are variety of herbal products that can be used to address worms and other parasites, but if you have these, it

is best that you are seen and treated by a physician trained to address these issues.

Step 3. MICROBIAL IMBALANCE

The bacteria in your gut play a key role in digestion. The location, type, and balance of the gut bacteria play a crucial role in the health of your gut and thus your immune system and your brain. There are two major issues to consider at this stage of restoring your gut health.

Small Intestine Bacterial Overgrowth (SIBO)

Most of the bacteria in the gut belong in the large intestine. When the small intestine has become invaded with excess bacteria, it results in a condition called small intestinal bacterial overgrowth (SIBO). Symptoms include heartburn, bloating, gas, and irregular bowel movements, and in severe cases you can develop weight loss and anemia.

Testing is accomplished by a breath test that measures the amount of hydrogen and methane in the air you expel into a bag over several hours after drinking a specific type of sugary beverage. Your physician can order this test. Testing for SIBO is available from:

Aerodiagnostics: https://aerodiagnostics.com/#service

Treatment can be accomplished with changes in diet and certain herbal combinations as well as antibiotics. Again, it is best to work with a nutritionist or health professional who is trained to diagnose and treat these issues. Typically, this would be a nutritionist, a health professional trained in functional medicine, or a gastroenterologist.

Dysbiosis (Gut Microbiome)

Dysbiosis is an imbalance in the flora of your gut. There can be many causes (medications, diet, stress, dysfunction of your pancreas or gallbladder), and dysbiosis can take many forms (yeast overgrowth, specific bacterial overgrowth such as Clostridia difficile, or an imbalance in the more than 1,000 species of bacteria that make up your gut microbiome). Remember, your gut microbiome is responsible for the digestion of your food, the health of your gut wall, and the health of your immune system and brain.

TEST: GI Effects
Genova Diagnostic Lab https://www.gdx.net/

This stool test gives us a great deal of information, including the balance of flora in the gut, how well you are absorbing fats in your diet, health of the gut wall, and inflammation of the gut.

TEST: Organic Acid Test
Great Plains Laboratories https://www.greatplainslaboratory.com

This test can identify issues with yeast or fungal overgrowth and gut dysbiosis. If you have overgrowth of certain bacterial species on this test called Clostridia, and especially if these bacteria are producing the organic acids 4-Cresol or HPHPA, they need to be treated. The two chemicals produced by these bacteria are neurotoxins.

TREATMENT

Depending on your results, there are different combinations of herbs, diets, and supplements that work for different conditions. Some of the products and companies we use are:

Candibactin AR/BR herbal formulas from Metagenics (https://www.metagenics.com) to help balance the flora in your gut.
Biocidin (https://biocidin.com) also for maintenance of healthy gut flora.
Dysbiocide/ FC-Cidal (https://biocidin.com) maintenance of healthy gut flora.

Addressing these issues can get complicated, and it is best to work with a nutritionist and/or a health professional trained in functional medicine to help you navigate the complexities of treatment. The Institute for Functional Medicine can help you find a practitioner in your area.
https://www.ifm.org/find-a-practitioner/

Step 4. SEAL AND HEAL THE GUT

Once you have addressed any parasites and bacterial or yeast overgrowth, you have to seal the gut. It is possible to do a leaky gut or intestinal permeability test, but if your bowel movements have returned (one to two formed bowel movements a day) without other symptoms of stomach or intestinal upset, skin rashes, chronic nasal congestion, or chronic allergies, you may not need those tests.
Genova Diagnostics Labs https://www.gdx.net
Vibrant America https://www.vibrant-america.com/

TREATMENT
Prebiotics and Probiotics
These are crucial for our health and all too often missing from our diet. Prebiotics are essentially fiber. Specifically, prebiotics are nutrient-rich, non-digestible fiber found in plants and vegetables. What plants and vegetables? Bananas, apples, garlic,

onions, barley, oats, asparagus, leeks, and dandelion greens to name just a few. Prebiotics are essential to good gut and overall health. They support the good bacteria in our gut, reduce inflammation in the gut, help to reduce the risk of heart disease by lowering cholesterol, aid in the balancing of hormones, and increase the absorption of calcium and magnesium.

Probiotics have been all over the news and touted to prevent disease and cure the common cold. They are the good bacteria that help keep us healthy. There are many types of probiotics, and each seems to play a different and important role in our health. Probiotics impact what we digest, the health of our gut, and the health of our immune system. The bacteria that appear to have the most benefits come from two main families: lactobacillus and bifidobacterium. Which probiotics to take and how much is an area of intense research. At this time, my recommendation is that if you are taking an antibiotic, you should also take probiotics: 50-100 billion CFU of a high-quality multiple strain probiotic to be taken with food and saccharomyces boulardii, 3 billion CFU twice a day, also with food. Saccharomyces is a nonpathogenic yeast used to protect against bad bacteria and yeast overgrowth in the gut. I prescribe probiotics on an individual basis and in accordance with the testing I have performed. Probiotics have been shown to be useful in treating irritable bowel syndrome, improving immune functioning, and treating constipation and diarrhea.

Diet is once again key. Foods high in probiotics include kefir, kimchi, yogurt, sauerkraut, kombucha, pickles, and miso. These may not be foods you eat normally so there is an argument that many of us could benefit from probiotic supplementation. Too much will produce bloating, gas, and diarrhea, so you may want to start low and go slow with the amount of probiotic you take.

Intermittent Fasting

When the body is deprived of nutrients, it shifts its metabolism to a state of rest and repair. This is ideal for healing a damaged gut. Be thoughtful when doing intermittent fasting. If you have chronic illness, such as diabetes, or you are taking medications for a serious illness, ask your physician if intermittent fasting is a safe practice for you.

My patients find that the easiest way to do an intermittent fast is to avoid eating for 14 hours every day. This can be achieved by simply not eating after 6:00 p.m. Break your fast the next morning at 9:00 a.m. and 14 hours will have passed.

Other options are alternate day fasting, weekend fasting, and restricting your eating to a four to five hour window every day. Intermittent fasting has been shown to not only help with mitochondrial repair but may also slow the aging process.

A 2020 study in the *Journal of Proteomics* evaluated the potential benefits of intermittent fasting. The study was conducted at Baylor College of Medicine in Texas. The scientists at Baylor specifically looked at the benefits of a dawn-to-sunset fast for 30 consecutive days. What they found should cause all of us to be very thoughtful about not just *what* we are eating but *when*. The study showed that a dawn-to-sunset fast:

- Increased a serum proteome protective against cancer.
- Upregulated proteins protective against obesity, diabetes, and metabolic syndrome.
- Induced key regulatory proteins of DNA repair and immune system.
- Upregulated proteins protective against Alzheimer's disease and neuropsychiatric disorders.[292]

We all know that food is medicine. What we are just beginning to recognize is that the timing of when we eat organic, nutritious food is critical in maintaining good immune and brain health, too.

CHAPTER 17

—

HEAL FROM ENVIRONMENTAL TOXINS

dentifying and ridding yourself of toxic poisons is essential for your recovery. In my practice, very sick people come to me who have not been responding to treatment. We often discover that they are suffering from toxic overload that no one had previously thought to consider.

It's always a surprise to me that doctors do not consider environmental toxins, since we all know that much of the food we eat has been contaminated by pesticides, antibiotics, and heavy metals. The tap water that was once safe to drink too often contains bacteria, lead, or pesticides. The air in many of our offices, homes, and cars is often worse than that of the world's most polluted cities.[293]

Treatment for all toxins that may be impacting your health is a simple process. First determine if you have a problem with mold toxins, heavy metals (lead and mercury particularly), and/or glyphosate (a pesticide). These are the big three.

We are exposed to thousands of chemical toxicants a day through our food, water, and air. I chose these three because they are common. Testing and treatment are unique for each one.

If you test positive for toxins, make sure you are not still being poisoned. Have your house, office, or school checked for mold. Test the water you drink for heavy metals, herbicides, pesticide, and other toxins. The air you breathe and the food you eat can be major sources of toxins. If the problem is that you are virtually living in a toxic swamp, we can't fix you until we get you out of the swamp. Then we can eliminate the toxins from your body.

Water

Drink more water. We are 60 percent water. Drinking enough water allows us to get rid of waste through urination, perspiration, and bowel movements. How much water is enough? If you are thirsty, you need to be drinking more. If your urine is darker than light yellow, you need to be drinking more. Ballpark estimates are eight, eight-ounce glasses of water a day, but some need more and some less. It depends on your size, your activity level, and your health.

A simple way to know your water needs is by dividing your weight (pounds) by two, and the number you get is the amount of water in ounces that your body needs.

Sleep

You must protect your sleep. One of the major purposes of sleep is to detoxify the brain.

Prebiotics and Probiotics

Prebiotics are non-digestible dietary fiber that supports the growth of probiotics. Prebiotics have numerous health benefits, they improve the health of the probiotics in our gut and the health of our intestines, as well as the health of our immune system and brain. A number of prebiotics have been shown to be beneficial in removing pesticides and heavy metals from our bodies. [294] Some of the best prebiotic foods include raw garlic, raw dandelion greens, raw or cooked onions, raw asparagus, bananas, and oats.

As for probiotics, some of the best foods are those that are fermented, such as kefir, sauerkraut, pickles, kimchi, and tempeh. Supplements are also available, and most of my patients are on pre- and probiotic supplements.

Diet

Ditch the junk food and eat clean. Eliminate processed foods and stick to organic and freshly prepared food as much as possible.

Your diet can go a long way to support and protect your liver or impair its ability to help you. One of the main functions of our liver is to metabolize and remove toxins from our bodies. Maintaining a healthy liver is critical to support detoxification of harmful pesticides, mold toxins, heavy metals, and even medications.

Limit the consumption of sugar-sweetened beverages and processed baked goods. Many studies have shown that the consumption of high fructose corn syrup (HFCS) is a major mediator in the pathology of liver disease, especially the Non-Alcoholic Fatty Liver Disease (NAFLD). [295] [296]

There are a wide range of fruits, grains, and vegetables that support liver health. Some of these include cruciferous vegetables (broccoli, Brussels sprouts, cauliflower, cabbage, arugula, radishes, kohlrabi), thiols (chives, scallions, garlic, onion, leeks), and leafy greens (chard, dandelion, beet greens, parsley, cilantro, endives, microgreens). Other foods that are liver and kidney detoxifiers include artichokes, asparagus, celery, all sprouts and berries.

All non-starchy vegetables and fruits help with detoxification to different degrees.

- Supplements for liver health can be a double-edged sword. Herbal and dietary supplements reportedly account for 20 percent of all hepatotoxicity in 2017.[297] Combination herbal formulas tend to be the most dangerous, and especially those containing anabolic steroids used for body building.[298] Nevertheless there are several supplements that might be helpful to support the liver during detoxification.
- Make sure you are taking a high-quality brand and the right dose. A little may be a good thing, but a lot may harm you, so do your research. These include Milk Thistle[299] [300] and vitamin E,[301] [302] (remembering that any vitamin E formula needs to be mixed tocopherols and not more than 400IU a day, as this may be toxic), Alpha lipoic acid (ALA),[303] and Dandelion root extract.[304]

Exercise

The benefits of exercise are legion, but one of the unsung benefits is the reduction of inflammation in the body and brain.[305] [306] I know many of you are struggling just to get out of bed in the morning, but this needs to be on the list and a goal to work toward because it is such a potent anti-inflammatory for the brain. Any amount of exercise you can tolerate is better than none. Also, always remember our mantra, "Pacing not pushing."

Antioxidant Supplements

Reactive oxygen species (ROS) are chemicals produced by our cells as they work to keep us alive. There is a balance in our bodies between the production of ROS and chemicals that eliminate the ROS called antioxidants. This balance is necessary for healthy cell function. When our bodies are stressed by toxins, pollutants, or even emotional stress, the amount of ROS tends to increase and can overwhelm our natural antioxidants. This is called oxidative stress. ROS are highly reactive molecules, and in abundance can damage our cells and organs. There are several supplements that can supply antioxidant support. These include liposomal glutathione, N-acetyl-Cystine (NAC), CoQ10 / UBQH, vitamins C and E, and beta carotene or vitamin A. More is not necessarily better, and remember that vitamins A and E can be toxic when too much is taken.[307]

Nicotinamide Riboside

This is a form of vitamin B3 whose mechanism of action is more complex than a straightforward antioxidant, but which specifically can help regenerate damaged mitochondria, the energy units of the cell. The brand I use is Tru Niagen (https://www.truniagen.com/).[308]

Drinking and Smoking

Limit or eliminate alcohol. One of the liver's main jobs is to eliminate waste and toxins from the body. More than 90 percent of alcohol is metabolized in the liver. Excess drinking can damage the liver and result in a fatty build-up. If you are toxic, why would you overburden your main waste removal plant?

If you are smoking or vaping, stop. Otherwise, read no further. You are just wasting your time.

MOLD

Mold is a nontechnical term for the fungi that grows in many of our buildings. The most common types of indoor mold are aspergillus, penicillin, cladosporium, alternaria, and stachybotrys chartarum (black mold). One type of stachybortrys chartarum is so toxic that it is used as a chemical weapon. Our concern here is not the mold itself, but the toxins they produce.

Remember that most people can process and rid their bodies of these toxins. About 20 percent of people do not eliminate these toxins, and the result of the build-up can be devastating.

STEP 1. TEST YOURSELF

Fortunately, we now have testing available to see if you have mold toxins circulating in your body. This testing is part of my standard workup for anyone who has been exposed to a water-damaged building or there is suspicion of exposure. The exposure does not have to be current or ongoing, because for those of you who cannot eliminate the mold toxins from your body, the toxins remain and continue to do damage to your brain and immune system for years.

There are two companies we use for testing, and sometimes, because they use different methods to detect mold toxins, we will use both to make sure we have not missed anything. In most states, you can order these tests directly from the lab and perform them without the need for a physician's order. Both of these tests are urine tests, so there is no need to have your blood drawn.

RealTime Labs: (https://realtimelab.com)
Great Plains Labs: (https://www.greatplainslaboratory.com)

I recommend that you take glutathione for ten days prior to doing the mold toxicity testing. If you have elevated mold toxins, the body tends to become deficient in the chemicals we need to remove the toxins from our tissues, especially the brain. Glutathione, which is the most abundant antioxidant in the brain, helps with the elimination of toxins and will mobilize mold toxins into the blood to be eliminated by the kidney. This will improve the accuracy of your test results.

There are other tests that a physician who understands the diagnosis and treatment of mold toxicity may perform. If these are positive, you have mold toxins in your system and there are things you can do for yourself to rid these poisons from your body.

Another test worth doing is the MTHFR gene analysis. The acronym stands for methyl-tetrahydrofolate reductase deficiency. This enzyme is responsible for clearing toxins from your system. Defects in this gene can inhibit or decelerate the detoxification pathways. One supplement I recommend to improve MTHFR function is methylated folate; it can be a part of a methylated B-Complex formula.

STEP 2. TEST YOUR ENVIRONMENT

Mold testing kits can be easily purchased at hardware stores or online. The ERMI test kit is the most popular. ERMI stand for the Environmental Relative Mold Index that was developed by the U.S. Environmental Protection Agency. If the ERMI test kit shows a very high mold index, you definitely have a problem. But if it shows you do not have a problem, the answer is less certain.

You may need to hire an indoor air quality specialist who can evaluate your home more thoroughly. I highly recommend that if you hire one of these professionals, locate one in your area who only does the air quality testing and does not also do remediation. This eliminates issues of conflict of interest.

STEP 3. TREAT YOURSELF

This can either be a pretty straightforward process or a bit more complicated. In the straightforward process, you need two things: something to increase your glutathione level and something to help absorb and eliminate the mold toxins from your body. There are a number of ways to accomplish this, but the short answer is:

1. Liposomal Glutathione as a pill or liquid and/or NAC, which is the precursor to glutathione.
2. A sequestering agent such as activated charcoal. We actually use a product called Ultrabinder from Quick Silver Scientific (https://www.quicksilverscientific.com).

The binding agent is necessary because the mold toxins that pass through the liver can be excreted into the intestine and reabsorbed into the blood stream. The binding agent traps the toxins in the stool and allows you to excrete them.

Remember that if you are taking activated charcoal or any absorptive agent, it acts as a sponge absorber of not only toxins but also medications, supplements, and nutrients. So, make sure you take all food, medications, and supplements at least one hour prior to taking the charcoal, or two hours after.

Follow this protocol for one month and then retest with one of the labs above. If you still have mold toxins, or if the amount of toxins in your urine is even higher than when you started, you are past the do-it-yourself stage and will need to see a physician who understands how to treat mold toxicity.

Three of my patients continued to be sick with very high levels of mold toxins in their bodies despite having their homes remediated after mold was found, each on two different occasions. These remediations can get expensive. Despite the remediations and my continuing attempt to treat them for their elevated mold toxicity levels, I could not get the mold toxins out of their systems. I finally asked the mold inspectors to punch holes in the walls of the bedrooms of these people's homes and insert a special scope to inspect behind the walls. This is not a normal part of the home inspection.

In all three cases, they found my patients' bedroom walls covered with black mold from previously undetected water damage to the homes. Once a third and more extensive remediation was performed to remove and replace all the contaminated walls, I was able to successfully resolve the mold toxicity issue in all three patients.

The other consideration in people who continue to have mold toxicity despite treatment is that you may be getting contaminated from some building where you attend school or work. Sometimes offices and schools will cooperate and allow testing of their buildings. On the several occasions when this was necessary, we found mold damage in these buildings and were able to get accommodations for our patients. Obviously, this is not something most schools or offices want to investigate for liability reasons.

If you still test positive for mold toxins after treating yourself and making sure you are not getting exposed from your home, school, or office, then the situation is a bit more complex. It is possible that there are bacteria in your nose called Multiple Antibiotic Resistant Coagulase Negative Staphylococci (MARCoNS). While the significance of finding MARCoNS is controversial with regard to mold toxicity, recent studies have confirmed that these bacteria can be the cause of chronic sinus infections.[309] In my experience and that of many others who treat patients with mold toxicity, testing for MARCoNS and treating them, if found, can make the difference between treatment success and failure.

The third major concern is that a chronic mold infection in your sinuses may be the source of your mold toxicity. This was demonstrated in a study by Dr. Dennis Brewer, who found that once the sinus source of the infection was eliminated, it was possible to eliminate the mold toxins from your body.[310] Mold toxicity is a problem that can and needs to be fixed for you to recover.

HEAVY METALS

Rather than expelling these toxins immediately, our bodies take the more cautious route of storing heavy metals, then excreting them slowly in order to minimize the potential for organ damage. But long-term storing or exposure of heavy metals can cause health problems, even if they are less dramatic than an acute reaction, such as that of a child accidentally swallowing a lead bullet and immediately being rushed to the emergency room.[311] Lead, arsenic, chromium, and mercury are extremely toxic, even in small quantities.

As elements, heavy metals are at least five times denser than water. The degree of toxicity is related to the degree of elemental density. Due to their high degree of density and toxicity, the mercury, lead, cadmium, chromium, titanium, and arsenic in our environment present significant health problems.[312]

Mercury

It is no surprise that the vast majority of Americans (89 percent) have mercury levels higher than the maximum limit recommended by U.S. government health agencies (below 5.0 mcg per liter.)[313] The average mercury levels in the population range between 2.0 and 89.5 mcg per liter.[314]

Lead

Lead can cause irreversible neurological damage, cardiovascular impairment, high blood pressure, decreased kidney function, and reproductive issues. Even very low levels of lead in children can cause learning problems, reduced IQ, impaired growth, hyperactivity, anemia, or hearing disorders. For children, there is no safe blood lead level. It should be avoided entirely.

The process for detoxification here is the same as for mold. Check and see if you have the problem. Eliminate the source if there is ongoing exposure, and then, if necessary, eliminate the heavy metals from your body. Many times, simply eliminating the source will allow the body to clear the toxic metal itself. If you need more than eliminating the source, then this last step is not a DIY. You need to be working with a health care professional who understands the detoxification process for heavy metals. If you do this process wrong, you can damage your kidneys and other organs.

> **TEST: Heavy Metals**
> These companies offer urine tests you can do at home:
> **Doctor's Data** https://www.doctorsdata
> **Great Plains Labs** https://www.greatplainslaboratory.com
> **Quicksilver The tri-test for Mercury** https://www.quicksilverscientific.com/
> **Thorne Heavy Metals** https://www.thorne.com/products/dp/heavy-metals-test

You can also get blood testing from Quest and LabCorp. The challenge is: what is normal? In essence, no lead and no mercury should be in your system. I believe that the private labs mentioned above give a better understanding as to how serious your heavy metal toxicity is if you have a problem.

TREATMENT
One particularly troubling source of heavy metal poisons can come from the very herbs you may be taking to improve your health. Heavy metal contaminates, especially lead, have

been found in traditional herbs from China and some of the Ayurvedic medicines from India.[315] In one study, 65 percent of Ayurvedic medicines sampled were contaminated with heavy metals, including lead, mercury, and arsenic.[316] I say this in no way to disparage Chinese herbal medicine or Ayurvedic medicine, but when taking any herbal medicine you have to know your source.

For lead, the most common source of ongoing exposure is water. Lead at any level is toxic, and while the goal is zero lead in our water supply, the EPA has as 15ug/liter as the maximum level that can be legitimately enforced and deemed safe. If you test positive for elevated lead, get the water you are drinking tested first. There are many companies that do water purification testing.

For mercury, the most common source is the fish we are eating.

- King mackerel
- Swordfish
- Tilefish
- Shark
- Marlin
- Orange roughy
- Bigeye tuna[317]

These are the most toxic and, in my opinion, should not be eaten. Unfortunately, there are many other fish that also contain mercury, though may be consumed in small amounts. Stick to these fish varieties: salmon (wild caught), mackerel, anchovies, sardines, and herring – hence the acronym SMASH.

If your tests show you have elevated mercury levels, stop eating all fish for three months and then recheck your levels. If they have returned to normal levels, then you have identified the problem. You can add fish back into your diet, but you must be very careful to eat only "low risk" fish and periodically check your mercury levels to make sure you are not getting poisoned again.

The other major potential source of mercury in your body is dental amalgams. Dental amalgams as a source of mercury toxicity is controversial, but there is plenty of evidence that they can be a problem.[318] If you have three or more dental amalgams in your mouth, you may want to consider having them removed. This needs to be done by a dentist who can do so without further poisoning you, or themselves for that matter. Typically, dentists who specialize in this type of care are called Biologic dentists.

SUPPLEMENTS

For heavy metal chelation, I recommend that you work with a practitioner who understands heavy metal toxicity and the protocols for appropriate removal of the heavy metals. The chelating agents (chelation is derived from the Greek word for claw, "chelos," so imagine the chemical latching onto the heavy metal to move it out of the tissues) may sometimes, rather than directly removing the heavy metals from your body, simply mobilize them and cause them to be redistributed to other tissues, creating more problems. The other concern with chelating agents is that they tend to not be especially picky about which metals they remove from your body, and so may also remove metals such as magnesium, copper, and zinc, which you need, and thus cause deficiencies.

All the basics I talked about earlier in this chapter for detoxification apply to heavy metal detoxification. You have to open the drainage pathway, so diet and sleep are critical to successfully fixing the problem. Fiber and good probiotics are essential. Supplements that have chelation properties include N-acetyl-cystine (NAC) Alpha lipoic acid (ALA), turmeric (curcumin), and Chlorella.[319, 320, 321]

Chlorella is especially interesting. Chlorella, a single-celled freshwater algae, is good for general detox as well for heavy metals. Chlorella is also highly nutritious and has been called a "super food" because it contains protein, iron, omega 3s, vitamin C, and other antioxidants and minerals.[322, 323]

ENVIRONMENTAL TOXINS

Glyphosate

The most common exposure to glyphosate is through the popular weed-killing product Roundup.[324] Several studies have exposed the detrimental impact that glyphosate in our diet can have on our gut microbiome and our brains in both human and animal studies.[325] The International Agency for Research on Cancer has also listed glyphosate as a probable carcinogen.[326] Unfortunately, once sprayed on crops, glyphosate tends to survive the harvesting and processing of the crops ending up in our food.

Other Environmental Toxins

As with all toxins, the first rule of treatment is to stop exposure. The Environmental Working Group (EWG) is an independent non-profit organization working to expose potential environmental dangers to our health in our food, air, soil, and water.[327] They have a number of excellent resources to guide you on how to eat healthily.

Stopping exposure is especially important with glyphosates and other environmental toxins because we do not have specific treatment to eliminate these particular toxins from our bodies. Unfortunately, the list of foods contaminated with glyphosate is very long. I refer you to the EWG website for a list of foods and the potential contaminates they possess: https://www.ewg.org/foodnews/five-lesser-known-foods-high-in-pesticides.php.

TESTS

Testing for environmental toxins in your body is tricky. Dr. Joseph Pizzorno, ND, has written extensively on environmental toxins and is one of the more thoughtful and creative people in the field. In an article he wrote in 2015, he cites numerous studies that suggest what we regard as normal results for our routine blood test are not but can be used to guide us in understanding our body's toxic load.[328] While these tests may point you in the direction of you being burdened with environmental toxins, they do not specify which toxins are harming you.

When testing for a specific toxin, you need to know what a normal level is, because some labs only test for the "presence" of a toxin or have a testing limit that may actually be higher than is healthy for you. The lab that I use for testing for glyphosates specifically, but also for a number of other environmental toxins that may have accumulated in your body is:

Great Plains Laboratory https://www.greatplainslaboratory.com/

TREATMENT

Although the impact of cumulative environmental exposure is different in each individual, the detoxification process involves similar steps for all toxins. It is not advisable to do it without the help of a qualified expert in detoxification, as other factors should be considered, such as nutritional intake and deficiencies, genetic makeup, digestive health, and emotional and physical stress.

A few supplements that help mobilize and excrete toxins are:

- **Apple cider vinegar** (contains bacteria that metabolize glyphosate)
- **Artichoke leaf extract** (enhances bile synthesis and flow and supports detoxification)

- **Humic and fulvic acid** (helps the body detox by replenishing the nutrient supply)
- **Activated charcoal, chlorella, and bentonite clay** (binds and eliminates toxins)
- **Probiotics**, particularly soil-based, spore-forming bacteria (facilitates metabolism of nutrients that support detoxification)

REDUCTION

To reduce your exposure to toxins, keep these tips in mind:

Fish

Avoid eating big fish, as they are more likely to contain high amounts of mercury. If you do buy salmon, swordfish, tuna or other big fish, always pay attention to the label. It should state clearly that it was caught in the wild. Otherwise, it is farm-raised and contains artificial food coloring.

Fruit

Obviously, whenever possible, purchase organic produce and/or labeled "non-GMO." Buy the freshest fruits and vegetables you can when they're in season. Wash them thoroughly under running water to remove pesticides and wax.

Add one tablespoon of vinegar to four quarts of water to wash your produce in bulk. Peel any fruits and vegetables that are not organic.

Containers

Avoid heating food in plastic containers in the microwave. Make sure all your plastic containers are BPA-free. Replace Teflon and aluminum cookware with stainless steel or cast-iron pots and pans.

Water Filters

Invest in a whole-house water filter. Pelican is a good option. Zero Water makes a reliable filtered pitcher.

Air Filters

Replace the air filters in your air conditioner and heater every two to three months. Be sure to open the windows for at least 30 minutes every day to allow fresh air and sunlight to enter the house, so it can kill germs and prevent them from multiplying.

Always avoid using air fresheners in the house or the car. Artificial scents in candles are often toxic, too. It is far better to use an essential oil burner to create your own blend of oils. Eucalyptus is anti-microbial and can kill mold in the air. It acts as a sinus decongestant as well.

Cleaning

Vinegar is an ideal cleaning agent. For windows, use 70 percent water and 30 percent distilled white vinegar in a spray bottle. For countertops, showers, and bathtubs: use 50 percent vinegar and 50 percent water, or sprinkle baking soda on a damp cloth, clean and rinse with warm water.

Purchase environmentally-friendly laundry and dishwasher detergents: Biokleen, Sun and Earth, Mrs. Myers, and Seventh Generation are the safest detergents according to EWG. org

Product App

EWG App and website make it easy to score your food and products for environmental safety.

CHAPTER 18

—

HEAL YOUR EMOTIONAL TRAUMA

Emotional trauma is an injury that is caused when we have an emotional response that is more than we can bear. The event that leads to that response may be so extreme that it would traumatize anyone. Or it may only traumatize those who lack the resources to metabolize their reactions at the time. In either case, it's the response, not the event, which causes the trauma.

This is extremely good news. It means that we have enormous power over whether and to what degree we are traumatized by events, whatever they may be. Not only can we work to recover from the traumas of the past, but we can actively learn the skills that will strengthen our resilience to trauma in the future.

It is in our nature to grow stronger with repeated exposure to stressors. Just as repetitions of exercises make us stronger, repeated exposure to emotional stressors can make us more resilient. Frontline trauma counselors who offer emotional support to victims of natural disasters, terrorism, or war develop the ability to modulate their responses to tragic events. Elementary school teachers whose hearts are broken when their young students say goodbye in their early years of teaching gradually learn to anticipate the loss and take it in stride. It is the same for parents who constantly fret over their eldest child in ways that would strike them as preposterous by the time the second or third child comes along.

We have a brilliant capacity to adapt. We may be thrown off-balance by an event the first few times it happens, but soon we learn to step back, put things in perspective, modulate our responses, and minimize the emotional trauma. We use this ability nearly every single day. If we didn't have it, we would not have survived this long. Yet life constantly finds ways to break our hearts.

Donald Kalsched, a Jungian analyst who specializes in trauma, saw a patient who was emotionally traumatized by reading about the horrors of the Holocaust for the first time. Without an emotionally literate family to offer her support and help her integrate the experience, she couldn't go to sleep and began to suffer anxiety attacks.[329] Films and video games with heightened depictions of pathos, tragedy, and violence can often have a traumatizing effect as well. It's not uncommon for a case of false memory to be traced back to a long-forgotten movie that had such an impact it was indistinguishable from a personal experience.

At any given moment in history, a long list of traumatic events are taking place – wars, terrorist attacks, ecological disasters, extinctions of whole species, hurricanes, tsunamis. The global pandemic of 2020 that combined social distancing and isolation with the fear of dying from a horrible disease was traumatizing to countless millions.

Physical reactions to trauma can somaticize the emotional trauma, expressing it as aches and pains, changes in sleep patterns, digestive issues, hypersensitivity to noise or touch, or increased reliance on alcohol or drugs.[330] Emotional reactions can include anxiety attacks, irritability, mood swings, night-mares, worry, feelings of helplessness, increased need to control everyday life, avoidance, depression, and denial.[331]

Many of these reactions are the mind's way of creating a buffer between us and the event that threatens to become an emotional trauma. Rather than feeling overwhelmingly devastated, terrified, or heartbroken, some people deflect those emotions, substituting a preferable state of mind, such as numbness or denial.

If deflecting emotions isn't enough to hold off the intolerable feelings, they may have to dissociate – disconnecting entirely from their feelings about or memories of the event. It is an extreme, but natural defense that is meant to protect us when our emotions become too much to bear.[332]

The trouble is that these coping mechanisms are only meant to be used temporarily until the crisis has passed. It is when they become entrenched that they start to undermine our health.

During the Vietnam War, water buffalo in the war zone turned to opium poppies to cope with the constant trauma of guns and bombs going off all around them, while many of the soldiers turned to heroin. In his classic book, *Intoxication*, Dr. Ronald Siegel, a leading psychopharmacologist at UCLA, explains that when the war ended and the level of stress returned to normal, the water buffalo stopped overeating poppies.[333] A lot of the soldiers, but not all of them, gave up heroin, too.

It is not uncommon for reactions that might have been a good stopgap in the short term to end up creating more stress for the body if they are sustained for months and years.

It's natural to experience a "fight or flight" response in the midst of a frightening, dangerous, or shocking event. The sudden pump of adrenaline our bodies produce is absolutely necessary for our survival in a crisis. Anger and fear can help propel us to take action or seek safety.

The range of potential traumas is nearly unlimited. Things like car accidents, domestic violence, assaults, sexual abuse, bullying, racism, identity theft, kidnapping, threats, stalking, trolling, unemployment, health issues, or the death of a loved one happen every day. As we've seen, we can experience emotional trauma vicariously by reading about a terrible event, watching a catastrophe over and over on the news, or even seeing a stranger attacked.

Yet some people continue to experience the trauma unabated. The emotional impact does not diminish with time. If anything, it grows stronger, burrowing into their psyche, impacting their immune system, and gradually developing the ability to destroy the person's health from the inside. When an emotional response to trauma begins to negatively impact their daily life, it can result in immune dysfunction and stress disorders that are linked to a significantly increased risk of autoimmune disease.[334] PTSD is also associated with cardiovascular conditions, bone and joint disease, neurological conditions, metabolic disease, and respiratory conditions.[335]

A high proportion (up to 80 percent) of people with autoimmune disease has reported unusual levels of emotional stress or trauma before they noticed the first symptoms of the disease. Once they have the disease, it creates its own trauma, resulting in a vicious cycle. That's why the treatment of autoimmune disease should always include the management of stress and emotional trauma.[336]

PTSD AND AUTOIMMUNE DISEASE

PTSD is a lingering response to emotional trauma that can occur immediately after an event or even many years later.

Most people notice symptoms within the first three months. In any given year, 3.5 of Americans will experience PTSD, with 37 percent being severe cases.[337]

The Diagnostic and Statistical Manual (DSM) breaks PTSD down into four categories. When a person has symptoms in each category for at least a month, they can be diagnosed with PTSD.

1. **Re-experiencing the trauma** through intrusive memories or flashbacks where the person feels or acts as if the trauma is recurring, disturbing thoughts when reminded of the trauma, nightmares, and intense physiological reactions (such as rapid heartbeat, anxiety, perspiration) when reminded of the trauma.

2. **Avoidance of reminders of the trauma**, including situations, people, places, or objects, and repressing thoughts or feelings about the trauma.

3. **Heightened reactivity related to the trauma**, such as unprovoked outbursts of emotion, self-destructive behavior, insomnia, and inability to concentrate when reminded of the trauma.

4. **Unstable thoughts or mood related to the trauma**, such as an inability to remember key details, blaming oneself or others, unable to modulate reactions of shame or horror, dampened ability to feel joy or satisfaction, and sense of detachment from others due to the trauma.

Although the DSM does not list autoimmune diseases and other illnesses as a part of its PTSD diagnosis, developing one of those illnesses is too often the next step.

Emotionally traumatic stress and PTSD may be identical in the immediate aftermath of a disaster or disturbing event. It is what happens next that makes them very different. If a person takes steps to actively relieve their emotional trauma and care for their emotional health, the trauma will gradually ease in time.

With PTSD, the symptoms don't subside within a month. The nervous system seems "stuck" in overdrive. It is as if the person is frozen in time at a place where the event is perpetually happening. The trauma does not diminish as the days go by. If anything, it gets worse.

Left unattended, PTSD can extend the pain of abuse in childhood, memories of war, and other emotional traumas for an entire lifetime. Studies done on the stress of childhood trauma show it dramatically increased the likelihood of hospitalization with a diagnosed autoimmune disease decades into adulthood. It can also provoke an existing vulnerability to mental illness.

RELATED MENTAL DISORDERS

The existence of other mental health issues can only exacerbate PTSD. More than 90 percent of people with PTSD have at least one mental health disorder. Depression, substance abuse, and anxiety are often found in adults with PTSD. Borderline personality disorder and antisocial personality disorder are also common. The impulsiveness of these personality styles may make them more vulnerable to an emotionally traumatic response.[338]

Mental illness is very common. As many as one in five adult experiences mental illness every year. In most cases, the first bouts of illness are visible by the twenties. But it can begin at any age and the effects may or may not be permanent.[339] The nature of mental illness is poorly understood, but its origins are thought to be primarily genetic or environmental:

- **Inherited traits:** Most common among those whose blood relatives are also mentally ill. Certain genes may increase the risk and trauma may trigger it.

- **Environmental exposures before birth:** Exposure to environmental stressors, inflammatory conditions, toxins, alcohol, or drugs in the womb.
- **Brain chemistry:** Impaired neurotransmitters (chemicals in the brain) interfere with neural receptors and systems.

Chronic medical conditions (such as diabetes or autoimmune disease), traumatic brain injury, a childhood history of abuse or neglect, substance abuse, traumatic experiences, and unhealthy relationships all raise the risk of mental illness.

The DSM-5 now lists almost 300 mental disorders. Anxiety disorders, impulse disorders, and eating disorders have become so familiar that they are almost taken for granted as a part of normal life in our culture. Among the other disorders, the most common are:

Trauma-related disorders

Mental illnesses related to trauma and stress used to be considered anxiety disorders, but anxiety is not always one of the symptoms. Sadness, apathy, lack of interest in life, aggression, anger, or dissociation are more likely.[340]

- Post-traumatic stress (PTSD) (lasting more than a month)
- Acute stress (like PTSD, but lasting no more than one month)
- Reactive attachment
- Disinhibited social engagement
- Adjustment

Personality disorders

As many as 10 to 13 percent of the population suffers from a personality disorder.[341] These disorders make it very difficult to function in daily life. They can be recognized by a rigid pattern of feeling, thinking, and behaving that is extreme. As in all mental illnesses, the degree of rigidity reflects the degree of pathology. Each of the disorders are very different, but they are each severe enough that they impair many different areas of a person's life. It is not uncommon for one person to have several disorders at once. If left untreated, it may be challenging for people with any of these disorders to take very good care of themselves. Illnesses are more likely to be ignored or go untreated.[342]

ASSESSMENTS

Mental Health American (MHA)
Since 1909, Mental Health America (MHA) has become the nation's leading community-based nonprofit dedicated to the needs of those with mental illness. It promotes early identification and intervention for anyone who is at risk. The website is a deep resource of very helpful articles on mental illness solutions and offers several online assessments.
https://screening.mhanational.org/

Mental Health Apps
https://onemindpsyberguide.org/apps/

MD APP
This site currently has 18 tests for mental health, including the Mood Disorder Questionnaire, The Homes and Rahe Stress Scale, Major Depression Index, Wender Utah ADHD Scale, Perceived Stress Scale and Hamilton Anxiety Scale.
https://www.mdapp.co/psychiatry/

Life Event Checklist
This tool checks for 16 common sources of extreme distress to help uncover potential mental health triggers.

https://www.ptsd.va.gov/professional/assessment/
documents/LEC5_Extended_Self-report.PDF

The Professional Interview Version is even more comprehensive.
https://www.ptsd.va.gov/professional/assessment/
documents/LEC-5_Interview.pdf

Minnesota Multiphasic Personality Inventory (MMPI)
The MMPI is the gold standard of assessment, used by mental health professionals to develop treatment plans. It should be administered and interpreted by a clinical psychologist or psychiatrist with special training in MMPI use. It takes 60 to 90 minutes to complete.

Million Clinical Multiaxial Inventory (MCMI-IV)
This well-regarded test assesses personality traits and psychopathology with 195 true-false questions. It takes 25 to 30 minutes to complete.

TREATMENTS

Whenever an emotional condition is given a label, there is always a risk of making the person feel discouraged and stigmatized. It's also true, though, that naming conditions can be very empowering. It allows you to take charge of your situation, get the help you need, and begin to make positive changes. Identifying your symptoms is often the first step to eliminating them.

It's said that healing is a marathon.[343] No magical treatment exists that will let you recover overnight. No particular form of psychotherapy works for everyone either. But with continued effort, determination, and support from those around you, you can find the right combination of solutions for you. Here are a few of the most effective solutions I've seen with my patients.

Eye Movement Desensitization and Reprocessing (EMDR)
Trauma can literally make changes to the way your brain works. EMDR helps recalibrate the brain's circuitry. In a treatment, you will be asked to follow the light of an EMDR device with your eyes from left to right at specific speeds before you discuss the emotional trauma.

Heart Rate Variability Training (HRV)
HRV teaches you to distance yourself from trauma by observing your physical reactions. HRV technology lets you know when your heart rate is too high, so you can deliberately intervene and use specific thoughts to calm your physiological response.

Neurofeedback (EEG Biofeedback)
Neurofeedback provides immediate feedback about your brainwave activity, then helps retrain these brain signals. It helps to alleviate various neurological and mental health disorders.

MEDITATION

Meditation is an integral part of the work we do with our patients. Early studies indicate that mediation has specific and beneficial effects on our first responders as well as our adaptive immune systems.[344] Meditation literally changes our brains and improves our resilience. It is also an invaluable aid in sleep, pain, and stress management. I encourage all of my patients to develop a regular mediation practice.

Two dear friends and colleagues of mine have written books that I recommend to all my patients. Dr. Elizabeth Stanley's

Widen the Window discusses her research on the impact of mediation on resilience in the military. In the course of a ten-week meditation training program, she used functional MRI studies to demonstrate growth of new neuronal tissue in areas of the brain associated with resilience. Her book explains the latest research on meditation along with her Mindfulness-Based Meditation Training program.

Dr. Tara Brach's books, *Radical Acceptance* and *Radical Compassion*, are especially empowering. She offers meditation exercises on her website and in her podcast. When we meditate, we inject far-reaching and long-lasting benefits into our lives.

How to Meditate

- Find a quiet, comfortable place to sit.
- Set a time limit.
- Close your eyes.
- Notice your breathing.
- Quiet your thoughts.
- Allow your body to rebalance.
- Close with gratitude and appreciation.

Forgiveness Meditation

As Nelson Mandela famously said, "When a deep injury is done to us, we never heal until we forgive." Forgiveness Meditation has proven to be very popular among my patients. Studies have shown that holding onto negative feelings about ourselves and others directly damages our health and blocks our ability to heal. Forgiveness demonstrably improves both psychological and physical health.[345]

That said, it is not necessarily easy to do, especially when it comes to ourselves. For that reason, forgiveness is more likely to take place over time than in one fell swoop.

The steps to the forgiveness meditation I use with my patients are surprisingly simple.

- Breathe deeply for several minutes, settling into a meditative state of mind.
- Holding the concept of forgiveness in your thoughts, invite the image of someone you know to appear and welcome them.
- Addressing this person, say: "For any harm you have done me, intentionally or unintentionally, I forgive you." Repeat it three times.
- When you feel a sense of acceptance or completion, say, "For any harm I have done you, intentionally or unintentionally, I am sorry."

It may well be that you have started the exercise with a different person in mind. You may forgive that person too, but always go with the one who comes to mind when you are in a relaxed, meditative state.

Our subconscious minds can process 500,000 times more information than our conscious minds (20,000,000 bits of information per second vs. 40 bits of information per second).[346] The images floating into your mind, as if by their own accord, are coming from your own subconscious. It is 500,000 times more adept at making choices than we are. Trust it.

The offense you forgive can be anything at all. Perhaps they missed an appointment and never apologized, behaved in a selfish, unthinking way, hurt someone you love, or neglected something you valued. The point is that you have held it against them. What you've held against them is of no consequence when it comes to forgiveness.

That said, it is always a better idea to start with smaller offenses. Deciding to forgive the most damaging wrongs you've ever suffered or those you are still struggling to survive is not to be taken lightly. The support of both a qualified therapist and your closest friends may be vital in these cases.

And it is always important to remember that "forgiving and forgetting" is not always appropriate. Abusive parents or partners may be forgiven, but inviting them back into your life for further abuse is both dangerous and misguided.

Your forgiveness is not for them. It is for you. Many people experience a deep sense of relief from releasing the burden of this dark weight. That physical and emotional relief is the goal, not reconciliation.

After reflecting on the process of forgiveness for this exercise, one of my patients said he felt as if he were trying to navigate down a river on a river barge connected to many other barges. All of these connections were emotional, but some were held in place by anger and resentment. They held him back and prevented him from moving down the river freely. As he tried to break loose, he realized they had been limiting him in ways he'd never realized, dictating choices in his life that he regretted, and affecting his beliefs about himself in ways that were harmful to his health. Working with the images his subconscious mind presented, he visualized releasing these connections to the other barges, allowing himself and the others to float down the river and find their own way.

THERAPY

Find a Therapist

Be sure to choose your therapist as carefully as you have chosen your physician. Because the bond between the therapist and client is so important, it makes sense to interview several therapists before making your decision.

Keep in mind that there is a significant difference between therapists. The term "therapist" or "psychotherapist" can refer to almost any licensed healthcare practitioner: a psychiatrist, a psychologist, mental health nurse, or social worker.

- **Specialist:** Certified in a matter of weeks or months to practice a particular form of therapy (such as rehabilitation, substance abuse work, EMDR, Reiki, or hypnotherapy), a specialist may have little or no other expertise in emotional trauma.
- **Social Worker (LCSW):** A licensed social worker with a master's degree in social work and 750 additional hours of supervised counseling out of 2,000 hours of social work. They specialize in counseling in schools and medical, government, or mental health organizations,[347] using strength-based theories to help people build on their best qualities.[348]
- **Psychiatric Mental Health Nurse (PMHN):** A licensed RN with two years as a full-time registered nurse and 2,000 hours of clinical practice in psychiatric-mental health nursing. They are also required to complete 30 hours of continuing education. They assess, diagnose, and treat psychiatric disorders with therapy as well as medical prescriptions.[349]
- **Marriage Family Therapist (MFT):** A licensed therapist with a two-year master's degree in counseling, or a related field, along with up to 3,000 additional hours of supervised counseling. They specialize in marriage counseling, group therapy, and family intervention using family systems theories.
- **Psychologist:** A licensed psychologist with five to seven years of graduate school for a doctorate degree, along with up to 3,000 additional hours of supervised clinical psychotherapy. They specialize in a range of disciplines focused on internal psychodynamics, based on mental processes and behavioral patterns.[350] They

are required to complete continuing education classes every year and are bound by the American Psychological Association (APA) to a strict code of ethical standards.[351]

- **Psychiatrist:** A medical doctor with a four-year residency in psychology for licensure. They may do psychotherapy, but often serve as the lead mental health professional responsible for diagnosing mental disorders and managing medications. They specialize in chemical imbalances within the brain.[352]

Find an APA Psychologist https://locator.apa.org/
Find a Psychiatrist http://finder.psychiatry.org/

TYPES OF THERAPY
COGNITIVE BEHAVIORAL THERAPY (CBT)
CBT helps patients change the way they think to make changing their behavior easier. It assumes that both negative actions and feelings occur because of our thoughts.

Therapists practicing CBT focus on identifying negative responses to stressful situations. Once the negative thoughts are identified, the person is free to behave in more constructive ways. Because it is so effective in certain situations, CBT is short-term therapy that is often successful in just 10 to 20 sessions.

PSYCHODYNAMIC TRAUMA THERAPY
Psychodynamic trauma therapy identifies the stuck place that the patient is struggling to move beyond. The therapist helps the patient determine what specific part of their response or interpretation of the event has so much emotional weight that it is interfering with their ability to process their trauma.

Emphasis is placed on insights into what the event means and why it is traumatic for that particular patient. The scope of the person's life is taken into account, including their childhood and developmental history, as well as their sense of self and their current relationships. Emotional and cognitive processing of what has been lost as a result of the trauma is a part of healing. The patient will be helped to release the trauma, re-integrate their life, and reclaim their strength and identity.

Regardless of the type of therapy they practice, any good therapist will come from a desire to help you heal your emotional trauma.[353]

GROUP THERAPY FOR TRAUMA

There are many different kinds of groups for people learning to cope with trauma. Therapists often offer group therapy for trauma survivors. Other groups are run by peers. It is always best to engage in personal therapy along with group therapy to make the most progress.

As Donald Kalsched, the Jungian analyst I mentioned earlier, points out, "We each live with a tremendous amount of loss and fear…about death, human limitation, the impermanence of life, what we're doing to ourselves, what we're doing to the planet. We desperately need emotionally literate and empathically-attuned containers with other people in which we can talk about the traumatic grief we experience, and to share it with other people. We need to form communities of like-minded people."[354]

At The Kaplan Center, because the emotional aspects of healing are so vital, I always have a therapist on our treatment team. Nothing can take the place of the life-changing dynamic that is possible with a qualified therapist.

The Chinese character for "crisis" conveys its meaning by combining two other words: danger and opportunity. Those who fully embrace recovery have the chance to experience unexpected benefits, such as inner strength, compassion for others, and a greater ability to experience joy and good health.[355]

CHAPTER 19

—

HEAL WITH SUPPORT

Almost everyone goes through a crisis," Jenn says. "Sometimes it's at the one-year mark: 'Oh my god, I've hit a year and I'm still not better.'"

Watching your friends check off the big life markers when you're missing them is another blow, she explains. Weddings, graduations, career milestones, baby showers, all shove it in your face: you've fallen behind. Your own visions of your future are nowhere in sight.

If you dare mention how you're feeling – not envious, not self-pitying, just sad and disappointed – people may sympathize, but they don't have a personal experience of your pain. Meeting with others just like you who struggle with the same emotions and are willing to share them in a group, no matter how devastating, heartbreaking, or embarrassing they may be, really helps. It normalizes what you're going through.

When Jenn started gathering together patients from The Kaplan Center for a single group, she had no idea how quickly word would spread about this invaluable means of supporting one another. Soon one group became many.

"We've got six to eight people in each group. More than that is too big. It means everyone doesn't have time to get to know each other or stay on top of what's happening to each other." That's why she ended up starting others. "We don't meet in person. We do video chats. All of us have brain fog issues. And that's fine. But it means that more people at once can be too much for most of our brains."

From Emily
As sympathetic as my family and other people are, there's a disconnect. They just can't understand. That's okay, but in our support group, there's a different level of closeness. I don't have to use as much energy to communicate with people who are also sick. We have a shared language and understanding.

It's a huge, essential part of my treatment to meet with this group. I don't feel like an isolated patient now. I feel connected to the others in a much more personal way.

FEELING UNDERSTOOD

The groups seem to work, really work. "Being understood by a group of warm, loving people; who wouldn't want that?" Jenn smiles.

"Even when we're just hanging out together at a café in town, someone might say, 'Okay, my time limit is one-and-a-half hours. Help me out, because otherwise I'll stay.' And everyone understands. People who aren't sick don't get it. It's like our common language. You don't have to explain."

It's such a relief to talk to someone who gets it. It means you don't have to feel like you're the only person in the world who is going through this.

Chronic illness is very isolating. Acknowledging that you feel alone isn't about feeling sorry for yourself. In fact, sometimes it's a struggle to confess it, even to yourself. So, it helps to be able to admit it in a group of friends who hate it just as much as you do but feel exactly the same way.

The important thing to remember is that this is not a therapy group. If members of the group need someone to work through intense personal issues, it is likely they need entire sessions with a qualified psychotherapist to make the best progress. Support from friends can be invaluable, but it isn't psychotherapy. Because there's a tendency for some group members to stretch the bounds of the group to meet those needs, it is crucial that the group leader set clear boundaries for everyone.

For those suffering from autoimmune issues, even regular socializing can be too much, so each session is relaxed. Everyone shows up in comfy clothes. A few bring ice packs after being poked and prodded at The Kaplan Center that day.

From Rebecca
We do it over a video call app used by The Kaplan Center. Only two of us live in D.C. The others are in New Jersey, Kentucky, Tennessee, and North Carolina.

It's so great to have friends who are going through the same kind of questions and concerns that you are, and you get a text saying: "Hey, has anyone been on this medicine?"

It's really fun when some of the out-of-town girls hang out with us in-town girls. We understand automatically what's going on.

There's wisdom, advice, emotional support. The biggest thing — besides not feeling alone, understanding what it's like to be chronically ill, and what a strain it puts on our families — is that I've learned so much about how to be gentle with myself.

I was really hard on myself for not accomplishing a task in a day or berating myself for various things. Then one day I realized that if one of the girls in the group put herself down like that, I'd be far more gentle with her than I was with myself. So I started offering myself that same level of kindness and it really helped me.

Sharing each other's woes and triumphs also makes you feel like there are people in the fight with you.

If health is like a five-pointed star, our group is a spoke on that star: therapists, doctors, nurses, old friends, and fellow fighters in the trenches with you.

You can lose battles. Nobody likes it. It's upsetting. But that doesn't mean you lose the war. Especially when we've got a great general and lots of trustworthy allies on our side.

LOSING FRIENDS

Everyone in the group has lost friends because they don't understand what it's like to be so sick but look fine. "If you cancel one too many times," Jenn says, "they move on. They feel like you've let them down. A friend of mine just had a baby. Everyone brought her food. She asked everyone to have a flu shot first. With my condition, I can't get one. But instead of understanding my needs, she decided I was unsupportive of her needs. They say that when bad luck befalls you, you find out who your real friends are. That's 100 percent true."

Of course, some people are naturally more empathetic. Others step up when they're exposed to a new situation and grow into it along the way. No one expects the illness to last a long time and limit your participation in their lives, so it can be hard to get them to appreciate the problem.

"Frankly, it can get tiring to explain to your friends and family, over and over, that you've got to go, even though you've only been there an hour," Jenn explains. "It's easy for them to take it personally, when you say you're exhausted and have to leave, especially if you look perfectly fine.

"Beyond that, they can't understand what it's like for this to go on for years and years. When most people get sick, it sucks, but it will end. How can they understand that you are literally not getting a break from this? No weekends off. No holidays. No rewards for good behavior."

The only break Jenn got from this was when she went to dinner with her parents and didn't talk about her illness at all. It's not that she was lying or in denial. It was just a relief to feel normal for a while. The illness is a downer, not a dinner conversation.

> *From Rachel*
>
> *Treatment for chronic illness is expensive, time-consuming, and exhausting, physically and mentally. All the medications have side effects that throw you off your game.*
>
> *Until a few weeks ago, I was taking 58 pills a day from 33 prescriptions. Each one is taken at different intervals under varying conditions – with food, two hours after eating, never with each other, etc. Try managing that while your mind is in a fog, and you feel agitated or sluggish because of the last pills you took.*
>
> *In our support group, we trade best practices: using a spreadsheet, setting up a system for a week's worth of medications in Ziplocs. Every tip helps.*

RUNNING A GROUP

When you're running a group for the chronically ill, it requires a very different mindset. There's a lot more to keep in mind than when organizing a group of healthy, vibrant people at their best.

Everyone is going to need a lot more grace. It is inevitable that attendance will be unpredictable. Despite how much they look forward to the group and even rely on it for the support they need, it's also possible for the members to have a very bad day and be unable to attend. So, it's important to be unusually flexible.

"I've found it's better to text than email," Jenn says. "Email is too much to process. If someone's having a bad day, they just don't answer. So, I let it go, then follow up later to make sure they're okay." Her advice is to set up these elements:

- **Every other week for one hour:** Every week is too much. Once a month isn't enough. After about an hour, you can see the strain on people's faces.

- **Topics:** The first group has been going for a long time now. We know each other well and can ask about specific things going on in our lives. We talk a lot about the challenges of relying on our families in terms of independence, physical help, and finances. In a new group, people tell their stories.

- **Notices:** We pick a date for our next meeting and then I send a text to the group the morning of the meeting as a reminder. With brain fog, it's not always easy to remember, even if you've been eager to go to the next meeting for weeks. I ask everyone to shoot me a quick text if they're planning on coming. It allows me to plan a bit and know who isn't coming.

- **Updates:** Lately, I've started sending an update afterward to let everyone know what's going on, even if they couldn't come. That way, we all stay connected and can support each other via text conversations back-and-forth.

- **Connection:** Even a little encouragement by text to remind someone they're not alone makes a big difference. When big weather systems come in, it affects us all. How good it feels to text someone: "OMG! I feel like crap today!" And get their reply: "Me too!"

From Jackie
We do video calls because a fair number of people live out of state. But when they are in town for their appointments, we sometimes get together. That's always nice. Even if you just see them at the clinic, getting an infusion at the same time as they are, it makes the whole experience a lot more enjoyable.

SKILL SETS

A support group can be invaluable for the skill sets each member shares with the others. It takes very specific skills to be a good chronically ill patient.

- **Noise Reduction**
  Noise is a big problem with 50 percent of the people in Jenn's group. "When we get together, our tips on the latest ear plugs and noise reduction strategies are like water in the desert!"
  Everyone shares new ways they have discovered to effectively advocate for themselves in noisy places. "In 80 percent of the restaurants I go to," Jenn says, "I need to ask them to turn down the music or move our table to be far away from the speakers. Often, I specify in the reservation that we want a quiet table."

- **Time Limits**
  Respecting time limits is essential. For Jenn, an hour is the mark. Experience has taught her that if she leaves in time – before her symptoms start to really spike – she is much better off. So, she has learned to honor that. If she can stop talking on the phone or reading or chatting at a

party before the symptoms spike, she may be able to take a little break, then keep going. But if she pushes past the time limit and they spike, she might be done for the entire day or even the next. It didn't come naturally, but she has come to accept these limits. It's better than the alternative.

Not only does she set these boundaries for herself, but she also tells the people she's talking to ahead of time that she will be leaving in an hour. That way, if there is any conversation about it, she can have it while she's feeling fine, not when she's on the brink of plunging into a crisis or feeling much worse. Sometimes it helps to remind friends that it's better to go for an hour than to stay at home.

Most friends understand and are not offended if you leave a party early, as long as they know what's going on and are not left to their own interpretations. But social expectations put a lot of pressure on all of us. We have grown up shaping our behavior to fit in and match the norm. It can take a real effort to allow yourself to respect your own limits and prioritize them above those social expectations. That's where having a support group filled with people who are struggling with the same challenges can make all the difference.

- **Personal Advocacy**
Learning to stick up for yourself is a challenge for most people. A support group can offset the fear that needing others to adjust to you in certain ways makes you selfish and "high maintenance." Nearly everyone with a chronic illness has worried about it, but those who have experienced the same problem know the difference. Protecting yourself while you're struggling with a difficult disease is not about being finicky or controlling, it's genuinely about guarding your health. When you're learning to

advocate for yourself, the support of the group can make it so much easier.

From Rachel

A big turning point for me began when I met an individual with similar symptoms and a similar history. The start of that turned into the support groups. This person is Jenn Sharp.

For the first time, talking to someone else with similar symptoms, I felt validated: "This is not in my head. I didn't make it up."

Even though the doctors couldn't fully figure out my condition, I'd met someone who had been through similar circumstances. The sense of kinship was profound. Almost like meeting your sister.

That connection was taken even further when our families were able to meet. Jenn's mom began to discuss the assistance Jenn required at that time (she had moved to DC from Michigan to help her.). Light bulbs went off for my mom.

It's not that she hadn't believed how sick I was or how much help I really needed, but it's very confusing for people when you look fine.

Sometimes they'll say, "Oh, I'm so glad you're feeling better. You look great!" when I know that I couldn't lift my arms to put on makeup, that my husband had to drive me to meet them, that I couldn't do laundry, so I had to wear whatever I had.

You're walking and talking, and you have a little color in your face, so they think you're back. But you're not.

After talking to Jenn's mom, my own mom said to me, "I am so sorry. I didn't understand. I haven't been there for you." So I asked her to read a few books. When she did, she began to understand. This is a family disease. Chronic illness affects everybody, not just one individual.

Meeting Jenn helped tremendously. Holidays are difficult when you have brain and body inflammation. The noise, the lighting, the stress of getting there or making food or buying presents crescendo for us on holidays and it gets very lonely. At least a few times a year on holidays, I talk to Jenn. Easter, Thanksgiving, Xmas day. We're in rooms with no lights, not able to watch TV. Our brains won't allow us to read. We can't be on the computer. So we're just hearing what everybody else is doing, but we can't do.

She's been a godsend. To have her acknowledge that, yeah, this is real; it helps a lot. In our support group, we share best practices, inspiration, and lift each other up. We share family issues, treatment, anger over our inability to control our health, what we want to do but can't, and help each other through it. Weddings and vacations, for example, can make our symptoms go crazy. Together, we talk about how to plan ahead. How are you going to rest to allow you to participate? What's your exit strategy? Where can you go for 15 minutes to calm your brain down? Do you need to take your own food because the food upsets your digestive system which is inflamed? Have you gotten those great earplugs?

We coach each other all the way through how many hours we can participate to still feel like you were part of it. Can you be there for two sets of three hours, or does it have to be eight hours? Then you can go to bed and not be upset about missing it because you at least got to go.

When your friends have gone through the same issues you have, they know exactly what to ask and what might help!

TIPS FROM JENN

At The Kaplan Center, Jennifer Sharp, affectionately known as "Jenn," has led the way in starting support groups that have provided connection and resources to all of their members. Although not all our patients live in the McLean, Virginia, or Washington, D.C. area, the members come to the support groups whenever they're in town and many keep in touch by text, email, or video during the weeks in between. All of them speak of their gratitude for her leadership and support as they struggle with a disease that few others have experienced first-hand.

Jenn is one of those rare individuals who has somehow found a way to reach out to others despite the magnitude of her own suffering. "I woke up as a senior in high school with a really bad headache," Jenn says. "Everyone thought it was a tension headache. But it's never gone away. I'm 31. I have had headaches every day since I was 17."

She spent five years struggling to complete a degree in architecture at the University of Michigan and finally switched her major to psychology. At the headache clinic, the doctors spent weeks running tests, trying biofeedback, EMDR, occipital nerve blocks and one medication after another. No one could identify the problem.

"I was popping pills three to four times a day to keep my headache down to a five to seven level on the pain scale. The frequency and intensity had picked up through the years. My choice was to stay in bed or stay up and fight through the pain," Jenn said. "No one had answers. No one knew either that pushing through was making my condition deteriorate. It sucked, but if there's no answer, what can you do?"

Finally in 2010, Jenn moved to Washington, D.C. She hoped that in a different city she might find some answers, but none of the neurologists she saw had any clue. A local physician renewed the prescriptions she'd been taking. Somehow, she survived on a barrage of medication from 2010 to 2014, but her symptoms continued to increase. Ultimately, she would have more than 50 symptoms and diagnoses, ranging from chronic daily headaches to occipital neuralgia, widespread somatic dysfunctions, irritable bowel syndrome, cervicalgia, hyperacusis, nausea, back pain, extreme constipation, chronic pain syndrome, dysautonomia, anemia, and many others in a relentless cascade.

Then one day, a close friend happened to mention a doctor in D.C. who had figured out a weird health thing for her friend that no one else could figure out.

"Is he a neurologist?" Jenn asked.

"No," her friend said.

"Okay, then I'll try him. The last thing I want is another neurologist. I've already seen ten of them."

When I first met her, it was February of 2014. After making a career of speaking to doctors for so many years, she was surprised that I spent almost two hours thoroughly going over her medical history, then ran more tests than any of the doctors she'd encountered. When the tests came back, the long list of diagnoses included an underlying infection: Lyme.

"I don't know much about Lyme," Jenn told me. "But I've read that testing can produce a false positive."

"Not this time," I said. "You lit up like a Christmas tree. You need to come in as soon as possible, so we can start treatment."

With a growing number of symptoms plaguing her for so many years, Jenn's road to recovery has been slow and arduous. Early on, I warned her that some of the treatments were likely to make her feel worse before she felt better and that has proven to be the case, but we are making steady progress, despite the ups and downs.

On her own initiative, Jenn started a support group for patients at The Kaplan Center who were going through similar struggles. So many women have wanted to join the group that she's now maintaining two of them. Everyone who attends speaks of it as a lifeline.

Through trial and error, she has learned what works and what doesn't when it comes to running groups for those suffering from autoimmune disease. She has kindly offered to share her methods for organizing these groups with us here.

1. Starting Your Own Support Group:

Group Size: You want a group that is between six and eight people. Any more is too many people. The group traditionally meets every two weeks. *(See "Structure" section for more details.)*

I've found the best time to meet is every two weeks around 2:00 or 3:00 p.m. on Thursdays or Fridays. Most chronically ill people do not function well in the morning or evening. *(See "Structure" section for more details.)*

The participants in the group should have commonalities in what chronic illness they are dealing with. While there are broader topics that most chronic illness patients deal with, to really get the most out of the group you want them to be dealing with similar illnesses (for example, all autoimmune, or Lyme, or chronic pain).

- Since they are most likely to be dealing with similar symptoms, – treatments, lifestyle changes, etc. – they will be able to relate to each other much better. \

As a facilitator, have a standard intro text or email to send to new members introducing the group, who you are, the purpose of the group, how often it's going to meet, and any expectations about attendance.

- Because people are chronically ill, they might not respond to you the first time even though they have expressed interest. Many times, I start with texting them and then send a follow-up email once we touch base with more details. But you might need to call or email or reach out multiple times. Don't get frustrated if you reach out to someone during a bad day or week; they might not have the energy to respond and then might completely forget you reached out (because they have memory problems or a lot going on with their illness).

The first couple of get-togethers will be "getting to know you" sessions. Everyone might not be able to make it to the first meeting. I usually ask people to give a history of their illness, tell us about themselves (family, job, school, etc.), what stage are they in their treatment, what are their diagnoses, and what treatments are they currently doing.

- Doing this many times helps participants find commonalities among their situation and also helps others to know what each other is going through.
- The second and third meeting might also have to be "get to know you" sessions because you couldn't get through everyone the first time or new people have joined. When that happens, since the group is so new, I have the people that haven't shared before go first and then if there's time, let the people that shared last week share some of their story.

- If someone joins a few months late, I do an abbreviated version of this with all the existing group members and have the new people give us their full story.

Set-up a Google calendar invite with reminders, so that it pops up on everyone's phones/calendars.

2. Lessons Learned

Send a text the day of the group reminding everyone that group is happening that day and at what time. Many people have memory problems or are not feeling well enough and lose track of the day. So, you'll get better attendance this way.
- I also sometimes ask them to let me know if they are planning on attending just so I can know going in. But many times you still won't get an accurate count.

This is unlike leading any other group; this is a group of chronically sick people. This means they might have to not attend/cancel because of doctor appointments or not feeling well. They also might be doing well until ten minutes before the call and cancel at the last minute.
- There will be weeks where no one can make it; as the facilitator you have to be okay with that. That just means you get back an extra hour in your day.
- This also means it's a sign that the people in your group might not be doing well. So, I traditionally reach out to check on people, even if they don't respond.

This is a chronically ill population; it takes a lot of empathy, patience, and understanding to lead this type of group. You cannot take it personally if no one shows up. It's not that people don't appreciate your effort or the group, they just aren't doing well.

There will be days that five or six people show up. On these days, make sure everyone is getting at least some time to talk. If one person has something they need to really talk about then that's fine; just don't let it be the only person the group hears from.

Also, when a group has five or six people show up, you are going to have to pay even more attention to timing because it will be easier to run over an hour.

It's possible that you will have group members that very rarely attend the bi-weekly meetings. That is totally fine, they can still be part of the group. They might be so sick that talking for an hour, even over the computer, is too much. They might just want to participate via the text chain or meet up in person when people are around. All different versions of people being involved are acceptable and you need to meet people where they are.

- If they drop off the face of the Earth for three months and then pop back up, just welcome them back in. They could have been having a really rough couple of months health-wise.

When things in life other than the chronic illness people are dealing with goes wrong, it throws everything off. Because most likely they are just holding life together from their illness. So be cognizant of the fact that some people will just need space, some more support; many times people's symptoms will flare up and they might need to be reminded that's why they are feeling worse.

3. Structure and Purpose of Group
Purpose:
- The group culture should be like getting together with your good friends for tea or coffee to chat and catch-up.

These are not structured therapy groups with specific agenda topics each time or reading/homework that is given each week.

- The purpose of the group is for people with common medical illnesses to get together and talk about the treatments they are going through, the actual disease itself, the side effects, what helps mitigate the side effects or pains along the way (for example, for Lyme, ways to detox), and how it's affecting their relationships with family, significant others, kids, friends, and other people in their life. It's also an opportunity to talk about what it means when you have to modify or leave school or work because you're so ill. It's a place for people to feel like they can completely be who they are and how they feel. Chronically ill people often are putting up a front for the rest of the world that they are doing better than they really are. The group is meant for people to be able to show up and say, for example, "It's a bad brain fog day," and have the peace of mind that people get it, and they don't have to explain every detail.

Structure:
- I would recommend that groups not be more than eight people. In any given group, you will most likely get two to six people that will show up.
  1. Any more than six-eight and you don't have enough time to get through everyone before people start hitting their physical and cognitive limit.
  2. Plus, it's too many people trying to talk and cognitively too much for patients' brains to try and track.

3. Many people will have memory problems, so more than seven other people to keep track of who they are, their stories, etc. will be difficult.

4. Plus, a large part of the group is checking in with each other between meetings (mostly via text) and you can't keep up with more people than that.

- I have found the best time to meet is every two weeks around 2:00 or 3:00 p.m. on Thursdays or Fridays. Most chronically ill people do not function well in the morning or evening.

    1. Every week is way too much and once a month isn't enough, especially since typically only half your group will show up at one time. So, this way you catch most people once a month.

    2. I did send out a Doodle poll to one of the groups to find the best day and time, so that is an option as well.

- We meet for an hour, and I try really hard to stick to that. That is the most people's physical and mental capacity can take, and I can usually see people starting to fade by then. You don't want the group to overly tax and push the members above their limits. Sometimes it is longer if someone really needs to talk, or people are having a good day.

- If someone needs to leave early because they are not feeling well, that is totally fine. Encourage people to speak up for what they need.

- Even though the group may start at 3:00 p.m., it's common that people pop in 10, 15, or 20 minutes late because they are moving slowly that day, had appointments, etc. That is totally okay. What's important is people are there. Sometimes this means things from the beginning of the group get repeated, and that's fine too, because sometimes something different comes up.

- I don't plan certain topics or structure for each group. Everyone that is chronically ill is getting enough of that in their doctor appointments, therapy, etc. Once again, think of this as sitting down to tea with your friends and catching up on life.

1. It's very common that people are cuddled up in blankets, drinking tea, eating, in hoodies, no makeup, sometimes laying down on the couch because they want to be there, but are in pain or tired. All that is 100 percent okay because it makes people comfortable and means they are attending.

2. I usually just start with the question, "How are you doing?" to someone or, "How is X treatment going?" or whatever, you know, they are going through. And we work our way around to everyone. Many people will need prompting to speak up. So, when there's a lull after someone is done speaking, I just nicely ask someone else how they are doing.

3. As the facilitator, you really don't need to talk a ton, just keep the conversation moving. Silence is okay too. Sometimes people are thinking or waiting to speak up, so don't try and jump in right away as soon as it's quiet.

4. There will be a common theme (treatments, alignments, meds, etc.) that everyone can

relate to and other times only part of the group can. I try and keep an eye on that and if someone hasn't been included in the last part of the conversation, try to find a way to pull them in on the next topic.

- The group is set up to meet every two weeks virtually. We have people from all over the country in our groups. But even if you were all local you still might want to do virtual (depending on your members) because getting out of the house can be a huge challenge for chronically ill people. And they will come if they can just turn on their computer and not have to use all their energy to get to a coffee shop. Plus, some of this information is very private, so people might not be as open in public spaces. So, if you are to meet in person, I would recommend someone's house.

- Getting together / Meeting up:
  1. There's the every-other-week meetings.
  2. We do try to get together in-person when people are in town for treatment. A few of us are local, so we are always here and can typically meet up. As the facilitator, I try and keep track of who is going to be in town when and coordinate the day and time we are going to meet up.
  3. We find it best to go to someone's hotel room, Airbnb, or home. This way everyone can just show up however they feel, especially if they have been in doctor appointments all day and they might need ice packs or a really comfy place to sit.
  4. Many also have noise and light sensitivities, so meeting at someone's place allows

you to control the environment a lot more.

5. Sometimes we do go out for coffee or dinner, but we try and be cognizant of where we are going so that it's comfortable and conducive to everyone's needs.

6. We also have a text chain for the group that is used very frequently. People will just reach out because it's a rough day and they need to be reminded they are not alone in this. Sometimes someone is having a weird symptom and they want to know if anyone else has experienced it and if they know of good remedies. Many times, we're reaching out because we know someone is going through a rough time and it's common that people, because they are feeling so bad, don't actually reach out when times are bad. So as the facilitator, I try and keep track of who we have not heard from in a while because that's a sign things are not going well.

4. Benefits of the Group (As stated by multiple different group members):
Combating isolation is definitely one of the major benefits. I have my own small group of friends walking the chronic illness path. There's a sense of comfort and consolation. There have been lots of times when someone has been unable to understand what I'm going through or times when I get so tired of explaining things that I think to myself, "At least my group gets it." That thought alone keeps away the terrible, overwhelming feeling that I'm alone in this fight, that no one can understand, that I'm doomed to be different. Humans crave connection and understanding. One of the worst things

that chronic illness does, one of the worst symptoms, if you will, is taking that from us. This group helps fulfill that fundamental need.

It also helps with practical things, like sharing symptoms and tips and tricks (helps doctors see patterns and connections). And it also gives us a space to feel like regular people again. We can talk and laugh and cry, share our triumphs and sorrows, and cancel at the last minute, all without having to explain ourselves. Because the group gets it. The group understands. I love that space. I need that space. It keeps me going. I draw strength and courage from you all. I can walk this road because the group is walking it with me. I shudder to imagine walking it alone. Again, I agree with other members of the group, there is something so anxiety-reducing when there's a friend in the doctor's office at the same time. It's so uplifting and cheering! And knowing I get to see at least Jenn when I come and possibly one of the other members of the group. It makes traveling to D.C. more than just traveling to the doctor. There are friends to visit! This also helps me feel more normal, reminding me I am more than my illness. Maybe because illness is a common denominator for us, it ceases to be the one huge defining thing. Ironic, really, since it's what brings us together. But that's a paradox for you. That's how life works.

I think groups should start to be implemented across the medical community. It's pulled me out of a deep isolation. I don't always participate, but just knowing there are people who share my experience, who I can lean on when I need it is life changing. And lifesaving. If I had this when I was younger and first struggling with my health, it would've been…. I don't have the words to describe how different it would've made things. The sharing of tips and experiences is just as important and helpful to my health as my doctor visits. Many times, I only realized I had a symptom after one of you talked about it, and I realized I also had it. I think the group can help doctors see links of symptoms and possibly diagnose easier. It changes the doctor office experience to have friends walking down the hall and getting IVs next to me. It lowers my overall anxiety.

I have done this for many years alone. Through illness I lost all of my friends. The only person I really had to lean on was my mom, and as much as she tries to understand, she never could. When the girls from the group started coming into my life...that's when I really started to see significant improvement in my health. Having other women in my life that understood and were going through this experience played a huge role in giving me the mental and emotional strength and support to continue to push through this thing every day.

Just knowing that I can text any one of the women out of the blue if I'm having a rough time and need to talk makes everything better. Knowing I'm not alone and there are people who care makes everything better. It also makes it harder to disappear into yourself (so easy with chronic illness) when you have regularly scheduled calls and visits where you know you're going to see and talk to your friends going through this.

There's some kind of accountability to it too...no one is ever judgmental, which is a huge relief because so many other people in our lives can be, because they don't fully understand this disease. It's just a group of people who will always check up on you whether you want to be checked up on or not. In your low times, you need people that will reach out because they know the signs that you aren't doing well, and they will help pull you out of the dark and hard places going through this disease causes.

This support group has had so many life changing, lifesaving benefits through our support of one another. The group keeps my sanity intact in this foreign world that invaded every aspect of my life: physical, emotional, financial, mental, spiritual, and intellectual. This disease affects all relationships, and the support group gave my loved ones the first real opportunity to meet others with similar manifestations of the disease. This helped both tremendously! While they struggled to understand me and what was going on with me in the midst of this disease, they were able to meet and see and hear first-hand the struggles of others, which helped them understand me and my struggles better. It demonstrated to them that the symptoms I'm experiencing are all really part of this disease and are as hard, complicated, and frustrating as they hear me talk about. They get to see beautiful, intelligent, and motivated women tell their stories. Stories that mirror the suffering and struggle I'm going through. Last, as a testament to the magnitude of support, this group is my "go-to" for dark moments, the highs, the holiday angst, and more. I love all the girls that are part of this group!

Chronic illness can be so unbelievably isolating and even when you have a conventional "support network" of caring family and friends, a therapist, etc., building relationships with people sharing a similar experience is incomparable. The benefits include emotional support, helpful tips and tricks that we learn as we go (for example, Sea-Bands and Alka Seltzer Gold, but also more obscure discoveries, like avoiding artichokes on disulfiram.) Seeing other patients' setbacks helps keep me grounded in the realities I'm facing or could potentially face, but seeing their triumphs also gives me hope that there really is a finish line, and we're all going to end up on the same side of it eventually.

Smaller support groups have a much greater impact – the controlled size gives us the ability to connect face to face (via Vsee or in person), really get to know each other on a deeper level, and the space feels safe and nonjudgmental. Larger online support groups are a whole different ballgame and often do more harm than good in the way they sensationalize certain treatments or topics without sound guidance of a trusted Lyme literate medical doctor, and cause an unjust amount of alarm and uncertainty.

Being chronically ill is extremely isolating
- If you are really sick, you can just be living day to day, trying to pass time and distract yourself from your pain and misery.
- Being chronically ill is the loneliest feeling I have ever encountered – you feel left out of almost everything because you can't relate; so I'm often loneliest in a crowd.
- It is so cathartic to be able to vent, especially to people who truly understand.
- On the positive side, with a support group, you do not feel as lonely, and there is a place where you are understood.

CHAPTER 20

—

HOPE FOR THE FUTURE

We have been wrong for years. Treating these new autoimmune diseases has forced us to improve our understanding of the immune system and how a misfire can cause it to turn against us. We are coming to understand that many cases of chronic fatigue syndrome, fibromyalgia, chronic unresponsive depression, and anxiety disorders, like the obsessive behavior disorder and rage attacks that we see in PANDAS and PANS, are symptoms of an underlying autoimmune disorder.

When an infection damages the immune system badly enough, it causes that part of us that is supposed to protect us and keep us in good health to attack us instead, mistaking our own tissue for an invader.

My first book, *Total Recovery*, focused on the innate immune system, the first responders to attacks. My work now is focused on the entirety of the immune system, including both the adaptive and innate immune systems.

In medical school, I was given what I now understand to be a very limited understanding of the role of autoimmunity in disease. We now understand that autoimmunity can be caused by an infection. The infection may be acute or dormant, but the infection, the vulnerabilities that set up the immune system, and the overactive immune system itself must all be addressed. Treating one without the other results in failure. Inevitably, the symptoms of autoimmunity emerge again.

As I sit here writing, I am thinking of a number of patients who have taught me so much in this quest to understand the nature of this immune system overload.

Tara was in excellent health until she was 22 years old. Shortly after graduating from college with a degree in dance, she was diagnosed with Lyme disease. Despite receiving treatments from a series of doctors, she continued to suffer from back pain and chronic headaches. Two years later, when she developed stomach pain and diarrhea, she was diagnosed with ulcerative colitis.

By the time I met her, not only had the treatment for ulcerative colitis been unsuccessful, but her weight had also dropped from 133 pounds to 98 pounds. Despite my best efforts and that of several gastroenterologists, Tara got progressively sicker. Soon she was in constant pain and weighed only 85 pounds.

When her parents heard about Dr. Thomas Borody, a gastroenterologist in Australia with a radically different approach to Tara's condition, she flew to Sydney for a consultation with an IV line in her arm, providing her with nutrition.

She returned with two startling revelations. First, Dr. Borody assured her that her diagnosis was not ulcerative colitis but Crohn's disease, an autoimmune disease that attacks the digestive track. Second, he revealed that the cause of her condition was an infection by a bacterium called *mycobacteria avium*. Dr. Borody believed that if we treated the bacteria, we could potentially cure her disease.

When she returned, we took his advice. After we eliminated the bacteria, Tara's other issues responded much more easily to treatment. We ended by working to soothe her immune system and return it to normal functioning.

Today, seven years later, Tara has married and has given birth to a gorgeous baby boy who is so adorable that my wife has repeatedly offered to raise him. Dr. Borody's insight was a game changer.

Infection Can Cause Autoimmune Disease

The concept that an infection can sometimes be the trigger that causes the immune system to turn on itself is not new. Many conventional autoimmune diseases, like Guillain-Barré, have long been associated with viral or bacterial infections. Multiple sclerosis, where the immune system literally destroys cells in the brain, has been associated with the same virus that causes mononucleosis, rheumatoid arthritis, and gum infections.[356] [357] Medical researchers have found a number of infections that cause the immune system to attack the brain, including the Epstein-Barr virus that causes mononucleosis, Lyme disease, and even the flu.

Several years before I met Tara, I saw a patient who had developed a gastrointestinal infection while traveling overseas. It was followed by such a severe weakness in his legs that he was hospitalized and diagnosed with Guillain-Barré, which is known to be set off by the *Campylobacter jejuni* bacteria that caused his gut infection.[358] Chuck was fortunate. Once the infection was treated, he progressively recovered his strength. He had always had active, physically demanding jobs in construction. Not only did his leg strength and usual vigor return, but he also started his own construction company and remains very hands-on in all his projects.

In 1998, Dr. Susan Swedo published a paper proposing that a common bacterial throat infection in children, Group A streptococcal infection, could cause a new autoimmune disease that attacked the brain, resulting in disturbing and dramatic psychiatric changes. Children suddenly developed severe anxiety, obsessive compulsive behavior, and other terrifying and disabling symptoms. Dr. Swedo called this condition pediatric autoimmune neuropsychiatric disorders associated with streptococcal infections (PANDAS).[359] When the condition is caused by other infections, it is called pediatric acute-onset neuropsychiatric syndrome (PANS).[360]

Dr. Swedo argued for a new type of autoimmune disease that physicians had been missing, leaving children sick and parents frightened and overwhelmed. At the time, these diseases were limited to children by definition. A PANDAS diagnosis in particular required that the condition begin before puberty, though PANS could potentially be present in adolescence.

I was well aware of these parameters when I met Nathan, whom you read about in Chapter 10. At 17, he had been an excellent student and a star wrestler at his high school. Then, six months prior to my seeing him, everything had changed. He began suffering from severe anxiety and an eating disorder. Strange bouts of sudden paralysis would come over him, leaving him unable to walk for days, then disappearing as suddenly as they arrived. This popular, gregarious boy fell prey to unprovoked rage attacks, where he would destroy the house – even shattering a plate glass window in the living room. Between the global pain across his body, his constant headaches, and insomnia, he was so miserable that he could not possibly attend school.

Initially, he was diagnosed with an anxiety disorder and eating disorder. His violent rages left some physicians wondering about the sudden onset of mental illness. In my evaluation, I found Lyme disease, among other things. We treated every layer of his condition, but when we finally eradicated the Lyme as the instigating infection, everything fell into place.

His symptoms subsided. He quickly completed a GED to catch up, then started college classes. To ensure that this condition doesn't return, we also treated his immune system itself, returning it to a healthy state.

Brenda was another patient who changed my thinking. When she was 50 years old, she regularly worked 60 to 80 hours a week as vice president of a major financial firm. That all changed when she developed severe headaches, body pain, and fatigue after a vacation overseas. She became sensitive to light and sound and struggled to concentrate. Before long, she had to give up reading, which had taken up a major part of her day. Not only did it make her headaches worse, but she also had to keep re-reading the same paragraphs, because as soon as she finished reading one, she would forget what she'd read! Unable to keep up her prior pace at work, she took on a less demanding position at first, but within six months, she left work on medical disability. Because the underlying inflammation was untreated, it raged freely and her symptoms began to cascade; sleep disturbances, nausea, diarrhea, abdominal pain, and soon suicidal depression were added to the list.

After seeing over 20 physicians, her diagnosis from a major medical center was fibromyalgia, chronic daily headaches, chronic fatigue syndrome, depression, and irritable bowel syndrome. My own testing revealed two infections: Lyme disease and mononucleosis. By now, I was beginning to have growing confidence that infections lay behind a new kind of autoimmune presentation.

It was heartening to see that, yet again, once we treated and resolved the infections and the issues that set her up for a more complicated infection, she was well on her way to recovering her health. Already, Brenda has been able to cook meals, socialize with her family, read a book, go on a walk with her husband, and travel. None of this was possible in the years she was ill.

As I looked more closely at my patients suffering from chronic fatigue syndrome, fibromyalgia, chronic anxiety, and depressive disorders, I began to see that most of them also had undiagnosed and untreated infections that had triggered their autoimmune disease. That infection was the key. I soon found that it was also common for patients diagnosed with postural orthostatic tachycardia syndrome (POTS) to have a pre-existing infection. This means that the number of people suffering with unrecognized autoimmune diseases may increase by tens of millions.

Autoimmunity triggered by infection represents a new class of autoimmune disease. The good news is that we have already identified a host of very effective treatments for the initial infection itself and the accompanying symptoms. And we know only too well that we can't stop there but must also take the time to return the immune system itself to normal, so it doesn't remain hyperactive and confused about whether its own body is a friend or a foe.

The bad news is that this insight about infections is relatively unknown. As a result, your physicians are unlikely to have heard of the concept applied in this way. Some may be willing to consider it and look for an underlying infection at the root of your autoimmune condition, but it is essential that they also work to systematically eliminate the other symptoms, then actively calm the immune system with treatments like those mentioned in this book, to return you to good health.

Most of my patients have seen countless physicians. Too many have been dismissed by doctors who did not know what tests to run and could not understand their disease. Indeed, a friend and patient of mine who once struggled for years with the diagnosis of chronic fatigue syndrome, fibromyalgia, chronic pelvic pain, and severe bowel problems has written a book in which she calls people suffering with these conditions WOMI and MOMI: Women and Men of Mysterious Illness.[361] Thankfully, we have come to the end of the mystery. Now there is hope and a clear path for recovery.

Exciting Advances

As early as 2020, the Covid-19 pandemic left no doubt that the United States health care system faces a growing financial and social strain in managing complex chronic diseases. Between 2000 and 2030, the number of Americans living with chronic disease is predicted to increase by 37 percent, adding up to 46 million people. Most alarming: 27 percent of children under 19 years old have at least one chronic condition, and six percent suffer from more than one. By 2023, as many as 230 million Americans may suffer from chronic disease.[362]

We need faster diagnoses, treatments that are tailored to the individual, and pre-autoimmune prevention. Medical science has already given us some of the tools we need. There is every reason to believe that research and analysis will enable us to find even more.[363]

The convergence of healthcare and information technology – especially advances in data collection and analysis – is accelerating research in genomics, immunology, microbiomics, and systems biology faster than ever.[364] If anything, the pandemic has given us a rare period of time when the best medical minds around the world are turning their collective expertise to defeating a virus that shows every sign of developing into yet another autoimmune disease. It may well be that this high level of research taking place with absolute urgency on an international scale will give us insights into the dysfunctions of the immune system that take us far beyond our current knowledge.

Even now, medical developments across the board are sparking unprecedented innovation in healthcare, enabling us to dream of a future where every person gets the right care at the right time, even before disease strikes. And for those whose immune systems turn against them, there will be faster and more powerful solutions than ever before.

ACKNOWLEDGEMENTS

The work that I do requires a village. I am blessed to be surrounded by a team of gifted healers who have done incredible work with our patients and taught me much along the way. Our incredible physical therapy staff of Pat Alomar, Jeanne Scheele, and Jessica Briscoe Coleman – they are not just gifted clinicians but innovators and teachers. Jodi Brayton, our therapist whose expertise in working with our patients and their families with chronic illness and trauma is invaluable in our center. Nour Amri, our nutritionist, deserves a special note of gratitude for her contributions to the chapters on gastrointestinal issues and nutrition. Rebecca Berkson, our brilliant acupuncturist and herbalist. Laura Elizabeth Dorsett blesses our center with her insightful yoga and meditation instruction. Dr. Lisa Lilienfield, my dear friend and colleague, has taught me much about women's medicine and hormone therapies and is an accomplished, certified yoga practitioner. The office could not run without the expertise of our Executive Director, John Doleman, our biller June Guzdowski, our front office manager, Denita Keyes, and my rockstar at the front desk, Kumba Gbakima. Nash Nortey is not only my chief nursing assistant, but also a critical part of the Nursing team that includes my co-head nurses Robin Harris and Nan Kinder, who provide extraordinary care for our patients and try their best to keep me on time. Robin also gets special thanks for her edits of this manuscript. I am blessed to be able to work with such an extraordinary team.

For the pioneering work that they do, the privilege of co-treating any number of patients, and what they have taught me in the process I owe much to: Dr. Charles Ray Jones, Dr. Robert Bransfield, Dr. Robert Mozayeni, Dr. Beth Latimer, Dr. David Younger, Dr. Sam Shor, Dr. Helene Emsellem, and Dr. Joseph Bellanti. You have taken my calls for help, endured my many questions, and helped so many people recover their lives.

My dear friends and colleagues in the Georgetown Department of Physiology who were instrumental is bringing together the conference on autoimmunity of infectious etiology we held at Georgetown in 2019: Dr. Adi Haramati, Dr. Hakima Amri, and Dr. Michael Lumpkin. I cannot express enough my gratitude for your friendship and support.

I owe so much to my patients who have and continue to challenge me to learn more and grow as a physician. Thank you to all of you who were willing to share your stories for this book and especially to Jenn Sharp for creating the support groups and her contribution to the section of the book, helping to guide others as to how to set up similar groups. The work you have all done on your paths to recovery has been incredibly hard, but you have done so with such courage and grace. I am humbled by your strength and fortitude in the face of great challenges and grateful for the privilege to care for you.

There are two women without whose talent and support this book could not have been written.

Donna Beech, with whom this book was written. It has taken two years and many rewrites to get it right. You are a woman of great gifts, much patience, and a truly gifted writer. I could not have completed this book without you.

Fran, my wife, to whom this book is dedicated, has been

an incredible source of strength, support, and wisdom for me. She has never wavered in her faith in this project and not just tolerated but has been fully supportive of my spending many weekends and vacations researching and writing this book. I love you, Fran, and I am truly blessed that you are my wife. Thank you to both of you.

REFERENCES

[1] Ed Yong, Immunology Is Where Intuition Goes to Die. *The Atlantic*. Aug 5, 2020. https://www.theatlantic.com/health/archive/2020/08/covid-19-immunity-is-the-pandemics-central-mystery/614956/

[2] A list of autoimmune diseases and their symptoms. *Medical News Today*. https://www.medicalnewstoday.com/articles/list-of-autoimmunediseases#skin-and-connective-tissue.

[3] Dinse, G.E., et al., 'Increasing Prevalence of Antinuclear Antibodies in the United States.' *Arthritis & Rheumatology* 72: 6. Apr 7, 2020. https://doi.org/10.1002/art.41214.

[4] Feldman, Bonnie. 'An Invisible Epidemic. When Your Body Attacks Itself. Autoimmune Disease.' Jan 29, 2016. https://tincture.io/an-invisible-epidemic-when-your-body-attacks-itself-autoimmune-disease-5738b699de12

[5] Ibid.

[6] Ibid.

[7] Levine, Beth. 'Autoimmunity Rates Are on the Rise in the United States, Study Says. Everyday Health.' *Everyday Health*. Apr 17, 2020. https://www.everydayhealth.com/autoimmune-diseases/autoimmunity-rates-on-the-rise-in-the-united-states-study-says/

[8] Ercolini, A. M., & Miller, S. D. (2009). 'The Role of Infections in Autoimmune Disease.' *Clinical and Experimental Immunology* 155(1), 1–15. https://doi.org/10.1111/j.1365-2249.2008.03834.x.

[9] McCoy, Krisha. 'Can Infections Lead to Autoimmune Disorders?' *Everyday Health*. Dec 2, 2009. https://www.everydayhealth.com/autoimmune-disorders/understanding/are-autoimmune-diseases-caused-by-infections.aspx

[10] Ibid.

[11] Ramondetti, F., et al., 'Type 1 diabetes and measles, mumps and rubella childhood infections within the Italian Insulin-dependent Diabetes Registry.' *Diabet Med*. Jun 2012; 29(6): 761–6. doi: 10.1111/j.1464-5491.2011.03529.x.

[12] Arleevskaya, MI, et al., 'How Rheumatoid Arthritis Can Result from Provocation of the Immune System by Microorganisms and Viruses.' *Front Microbiol*. 2016; 7: 1296. doi: 10.3389/fmicb.2016.01296 https://www.ncbi.nlm.nih.gov/pmc/articles/PMC4987382/

[13] McCoy, Krisha. Ibid.

[14] McNees, A. et al., 'Mycobacterium paratuberculosis as a cause of Crohn's disease.' Expert Rev Gastroenterol Hepatol. . 2015;9(12):1523-34. doi: 10.1586/17474124.2015.1093931. Epub 2015 Oct 16. https://pubmed.ncbi.nlm.nih.gov/26474349/

[15] DOI: 10.1056/NEJM199511233332102

[16] Ercolini, A. M., & Miller, S. D. (2009). 'The role of infections in autoimmune disease.' *Clinical and Experimental Immunology* 155(1): 1–15. https://doi.org/10.1111/j.1365-2249.2008.03834.x

[17] Arango MT, Shoenfeld Y, Cervera R, et al. 'Infection and autoimmune diseases.' In Anaya JM, Shoenfeld Y, Rojas-Villarraga A, et al. (eds). *Autoimmunity: From Bench to Bedside* [Internet]. Bogota (Colombia): El Rosario University Press; 2013 Jul 18. Chapter 19. Available from: https://www.ncbi.nlm.nih.gov/books/NBK459437/.

[18] ADRESS LATER: Confirm footnotes for Chapter 2.There are two different sets. 12/20 Feldman, Bonnie. Ibid.

[19] Feldman, Bonnie. Ibid.

[20] Naviaux, Robert K. 'Metabolic features of the cell danger response.' *Mitochondrion* 16. May 2014, 7–17. https://doi.org/10.1016/j.mito.2013.08.006

[21] 'Study Guide to the Systems of the Body.' *ACLA Training Center*. Jul 13, 2019. https://www.acls.net/study-guide-body-systems.htm

[22] Tanya Lewis, 'Human Brain: Facts, Functions & Anatomy.' *LiveScience*. Sept 28, 2018. https://www.livescience.com/29365-human-brain.html

[23] '10 Interesting Facts About The Human Brain.' *ScienceFirst*. https://sciencefirst.com/10-interesting-facts-about-the-human-brain/

[24] Ann Brown. 'How Many Breaths Do You Take Each Day?' Environmental Protection Agency. https://blog.epa.gov/2014/04/28/how-many-breaths-do-you-take-each-day/

[25] 'How Many Heartbeats Do We Get?' U.S. Healthworks. Sept 19, 2011. https://www.ushealthworks.com/blog/2011/09/just-how-many-heartbeats-do-we-get/index.html

[26] Autoimmune Diseases. Office of Women's Health. U.S. Department of Health & Human Services. https://www.womenshealth.gov/a-z-topics/autoimmune-diseases

[27] 'Horror autotoxicus.' https://de.wikipedia.org/wiki/Horror_autotoxicus

[28] P. Valent, B. Groner, et al (March 2016). 'Paul Ehrlich (1854-1915) and His Contributions to the Foundation and Birth of Translational Medicine.' *Journal of Innate Immunity* 8 (1): 111–20. https://doi.org/10.1159/000443526 ; https://www.karger.com/Article/FullText/443526.

[29] Felix Bosch, Laia Rosich. 'The Contributions of Paul Ehrlich to Pharmacology: A Tribute on the Occasion of the Centenary of His Nobel Prize.' *Pharmacology.* 2008 Oct; 82(3): 171–179. doi: 10.1159/000149583 https://www.ncbi.nlm.nih.gov/pmc/articles/PMC2790789/.

[30] A. Silverstein. 'Horror autotoxicus, Autoimmunity and Immunoregulation: The Early History.' *Transfus Med Hemother* 2005. 32 (6): 296–302. https://www.karger.com/Article/PDF/89116.

[31] Opioid Overdose Crisis. National Institute on Drug Abuse. Jan 2019. https://www.drugabuse.gov/drugs-abuse/opioids/opioid-overdose-crisis.

[32] Afrin, Lawrence B., et al., 'Characterization of Mast Cell Activation Syndrome.' *Am J Med Sci.* 2017 Mar; 353(3): 207–215. doi: 10.1016/j.amjms.2016.12.013. Epub 2016 Dec 16. PMID: 28262205.

[33] Włodarczyk, M., Druszczyńska, M., & Fol, M. (2019). Trained Innate Immunity Not Always Amicable. *International Journal of Molecular Sciences* 20 (10): 2565. https://doi.org/10.3390/ijms20102565

[34] Celiac disease. National Center for Advancing Translational Sciences. https://rarediseases.info.nih.gov/diseases/11998/celiac-disease/cases/43805.

[35] Kuenstner, JT, et al., 'The Consensus from the Mycobacterium avium ssp. paratuberculosis (MAP) Conference 2017.' *Front Public Health.* 2017 Sep 27; 5: 208. doi: 10.3389/fpubh.2017.00208. eCollection 2017. PMID: 29021977

[36] Tarlinton, RE, et al., 'The Interaction between Viral and Environmental Risk Factors in the Pathogenesis of Multiple Sclerosis.' *Int J Mol Sci.* 2019 Jan 14; 20(2): 303. doi: 10.3390/ijms20020303. PMID: 30646507.

[37] Miller GE, Chen E, Parker KJ. 'Psychological stress in childhood and susceptibility to the chronic diseases of aging: moving

toward a model of behavioral and biological mechanisms.' *Psychological Bulletin*. 2011 Nov; 137(6): 959–97. DOI: 10.1037/a0024768. PMID: 21787044

[38] Ibid.

[39] Autoimmune Disease and Your Environment. National Institute of Environmental Health Sciences. April 2020. https://www.niehs.nih.gov/health/materials/autoimmune_diseases_508.pdf

[40] Ramey, Sarah. *The Lady's Handbook for Her Mysterious Illness* (Knopf Doubleday, 2019), p. 10.

[41] Wu, Katherine. 'Scientists Uncover Biological Signatures of the Worst Covid-19 Cases.' *New York Times*, Aug 4, 2020. https://www.nytimes.com/2020/08/04/health/coronavirus-immune-system.html?action=click&algo=top_conversion&block=trending_recirc&fellback=false&imp_id=.

[42] Ibid.

[43] Ibid.

[44] M. Rojas, P. Restrepo-Jiménez, D.M. Monsalve, et al., 'Molecular mimicry and autoimmunity.' *Journal of Autoimmunity* 95, December 2018, pp. 100–23. https://www.sciencedirect.com/science/article/pii/S0896841118305365.

[45] 'It's not ALL in the genes—the role of epigenetics.' Australian Academy of Science. https://www.science.org.au/curious/epigenetics.

[46] Niller HH, Wolf H, Ay E, Minarovits J. 'Epigenetic dysregulation of epstein-barr virus latency and development of autoimmune disease.' *Adv Exp Med Biol*. 2011; 711: 82–102. doi:10.1007/978-1-4419-8216-2_7.

[47] Ray D, Yung R. 'Immune senescence, epigenetics and autoimmunity.' *Clin Immunol*. 2018; 196: 59–63. doi:10.1016/j.clim.2018.04.002.

[48] Rudenko N, Golovchenko M, Kybicova K, Vancova M. 'Metamorphoses of Lyme disease spirochetes: phenomenon of Borrelia persisters.' *Parasite Vectors*. 2019; 12(1): 237. Published 2019, May 16. doi:10.1186/s13071-019-3495-7.

[49] Muhsin, Jamal, et. al. 'Bacterial biofilm and associated infections.' *Journal of the Chinese Medical Association* Jan 2018; 81(1): 7–11. https://doi.org/10.1016/j.jcma.2017.07.012.

[50] How many people get Lyme disease? Centers for Disease Control and Prevention, National Center for Emerging and Zoonotic

Infectious Diseases (NCEZID), Division of Vector-Borne Diseases (DVBD). Dec 21, 2018. https://www.cdc.gov/lyme/stats/human-cases.html.

[51] 'Transmission.' Centers for Disease Control and Prevention, National Center for Emerging and Zoonotic Infectious Diseases (NCEZID), Division of Vector-Borne Diseases (DVBD). Jan 29, 2020. https://www.cdc.gov/lyme/transmission/index.html.

[52] 'What you need to know about Borrelia mayonii.' Centers for Disease Control and Prevention, National Center for Emerging and Zoonotic Infectious Diseases (NCEZID), Division of Vector-Borne Diseases (DVBD). Sept 12, 2019. https://www.cdc.gov/lyme/mayonii/index.html.

[53] 'Factsheet about Borreliosis.' European Centre for Disease Prevention and Control. Mar 6, 2016. https://www.ecdc.europa.eu/en/borreliosis/facts/factsheet.

[54] Ticks. Lyme and Tick-Borne Diseases Research Center, Columbia University Irving Medical Center. https://www.columbia-lyme.org/faq.

[55] Kristoferitsch W, Aboulenein-Djamshidian F, Jecel J, et al. 'Secondary dementia due to Lyme neuroborreliosis.' *Wien Klin Wochenschr.* 2018; 130(15–16): 468–78. doi:10.1007/s00508-018-1361-9.

[56] Bransfield RC. 'The psychoimmunology of lyme/tick-borne diseases and its association with neuropsychiatric symptoms.' *Open Neurol J.* 2012; 6: 88–93. doi:10.2174/1874205X01206010088.

[57] Chang K, Frankovich J, Cooperstock M, et al. 'Clinical evaluation of youth with pediatric acute-onset neuropsychiatric syndrome (PANS): recommendations from the 2013 PANS Consensus Conference.' *J Child Adolesc Psychopharmacol.* 2015; 25(1): 3–13. doi:10.1089/cap.2014.0084.

[58] Ben-Harari, Ruben R. 'Tick transmission of toxoplasmosis.' *Journal Expert Review of Anti-infective Therapy* 17: 11, Oct 17, 2019. https://doi.org/10.1080/14787210.2019.1682550.

[59] Berghoff W. 'Chronic Lyme Disease and Co-infections: Differential Diagnosis.' *Open Neurol J.* 2012; 6: 158–178. doi:10.2174/1874205X01206010158.

[60] Knapp KL, Rice NA. 'Human Coinfection with Borrelia burgdorferi and Babesia microti in the United States.' *J Parasitol Res.* 2015; 587131. doi:10.1155/2015/587131.

[61] Bloomberg J, Rizwan M, Böhlin-Wiener A, et al. 'Antibodies to Human Herpesviruses in Myalgic Encephalomyelitis/Chronic Fatigue Syndrome Patients.' *Front Immunol.* 2019; 10: 1946. Published 2019, Aug 14. doi:10.3389/fimmu.2019.0194.

[62] Harley, John B. 'Transcription factors operate across disease loci, with EBNA2 implicated in autoimmunity.' *Nat Genet.* 2018; 50: 699–707. https://doi.org/10.1038/s41588-018-0102-3.

[63] Parrott, Gretchen, et al., 'A Compendium for Mycoplasma pneumoniae. Front.' *Microbiol*, April 12, 2016. https://doi.org/10.3389/fmicb.2016.00513.

[64] Nicholson, GL, et al., 'The Role of Chronic Bacterial and Viral Infections in Neurodegenerative, Neurobehavioral, Psychiatric, Autoimmune and Fatiguing Illnesses, Part 2.' *BJMP.* Mar 2010; 3: 1. https://www.bjmp.org/files/2010-3-1/bjmp-2010-3-1-301.pdf.

[65] Bajantri B, Venkatram S, Diaz-Fuentes G. '*Mycoplasma pneumoniae*: A Potentially Severe Infection.' *J Clin Med Res.* 2018;10(7): 535–44. doi:10.14740/jocmr3421w.

[66] 'What is Sleep? Why is it needed?' American Sleep Association. https://www.sleepassociation.org/about-sleep/what-is-sleep/.

[67] Da Mesquita, Sandro, et al., 'Functional aspects of meningeal lymphatics in ageing and Alzheimer's disease.' *Nature* 560, 185–91 (2018). https://doi.org/10.1038/s41586-018-0368-8.

[68] Absinta, Martina, et al., 'Human and nonhuman primate meninges harbor lymphatic vessels that can be visualized noninvasively by MRI.' *eLife* 2017; 6: e29738 DOI: 10.7554/eLife.29738.

[69] 'What is Sleep? Why is it needed?' American Sleep Association. https://www.sleepassociation.org/about-sleep/what-is-sleep/.

[70] Ibid.

[71] Ibid.

[72] Paul Bergner. 'Sleep Debt: Pathophysiology and Natural Therapeutics.' Medicines from the Earth 2008. https://www.botanical-medicine.org/index.php?route=product/product&product_id=1563.

[73] 'What is Sleep?'

[74] Paul Bergner.

[75] What is Sleep?

[76] Ibarra-Coronado, E. G., Pantaleón-Martínez, A. M., et al., 'The Bidirectional Relationship between Sleep and Immunity against Infections.' *Journal of Immunology Research*, 2015, 678164. https://doi.org/10.1155/2015/678164.

[77] Ibarra-Coronado, E. G., Pantaleón-Martínez, A. M., et al., 'The Bidirectional Relationship between Sleep and Immunity against Infections.' *Journal of Immunology Research*, 2015, 678164. https://doi.org/10.1155/2015/678164.

[78] Ibarra-Coronado, E. G., Pantaleón-Martínez, A. M., et al., 'The Bidirectional Relationship between Sleep and Immunity against Infections.' *Journal of Immunology Research*, 2015, 678164. https://doi.org/10.1155/2015/678164.

[79] Ibarra-Coronado, E. G., Pantaleón-Martínez, A. M., et al., 'The Bidirectional Relationship between Sleep and Immunity against Infections.' *Journal of Immunology Research*, 2015, 678164. https://doi.org/10.1155/2015/678164.

[80] Ibarra-Coronado, E. G., Pantaleón-Martínez, A. M., et al., 'The Bidirectional Relationship between Sleep and Immunity against Infections.' *Journal of Immunology Research*, 2015, 678164. https://doi.org/10.1155/2015/678164

[81] Irwin, Michael R. 'Why sleep is important for health: a psychoneuroimmunology perspective?' *Annu Rev Psychol*. Jan 3, 2015; 66:143–72. doi: 10.1146/annurev-psych-010213-115205. PMID:25061767.

[82] Olson, Eric, M.D., 'Lack of Sleep: Can It Make You Sick?' Mayo Clinic. https://www.mayoclinic.org/diseases-conditions/insomnia/expert-answers/lack-of-sleep/faq-20057757#:~:text=Yes%2C%20lack%20of%20sleep%20can,if%20you%20do%20get%20sick.

[83] Hsaio, Yi-Han, et al., 'Sleep disorders and increased risk of autoimmune diseases in individuals without sleep apnea.' *Sleep*. 2015, Apr 1; 38(4): 581–6. doi: 10.5665/sleep.4574 PMID:25669189.

[84] Haspel JA, Anafi R, Brown MK, et al. 'Perfect timing: circadian rhythms, sleep, and immunity - an NIH workshop summary.' *JCI Insight*. 2020, Jan 16; 5(1): e131487. doi:10.1172/jci.insight.131487.

[85] Paul Bergner. 'Sleep Debt: Pathophysiology and Natural Therapeutics.' Medicines from the Earth 2008. https://www.botanical-medicine.org/index.php?route=product/product&product_id=1563.

[86] PMID:25061767.

[87] Paul Bergner.

[88] Paul Bergner.

[89] Paul Bergner.

[90] Paul Bergner.

[91] 'What is "normal" sleep?' InformedHealth.org. Institute of Quality and Efficiency in Health Care. Sept 18, 2013. last update: December 30, 2016. https://www.ncbi.nlm.nih.gov/books/NBK279322/.

[92] 'What is "normal" sleep?'

[93] 'One in four Americans develop insomnia each year: 75% of them recover. University of Pennsylvania School of Medicine,' *ScienceDaily*. June 5, 2018. https://www.sciencedaily.com/releases/2018/06/180605154114.htm.

[94] 'A Very Short Course on Sleep Apnea.' *SleepApnea.org*. https://www.sleepapnea.org/learn/sleep-apnea-information-clinicians/.

[95] 'Narcolepsy Fast Facts.' Narcolepsy Network. https://narcolepsynetwork.org/about-narcolepsy/narcolepsy-fast-facts/.

[96] 'Judgment and Safety. Get Sleep.' Division of Sleep Medicine at Harvard Medical School http://healthysleep.med.harvard.edu/needsleep/whats-in-it-for-you/judgment-safety#top

[97] Ibid.

[98] Xie, Hong. 'Differential expression of immune markers in the patients with obstructive sleep apnea/hypopnea syndrome.' *Eur Arch Otorhinolaryngol*. 2019 Mar; 276(3): 735–44. doi: 10.1007/s00405-018-5219-6. Epub 2018 Dec 18. PMID:30560392.

[99] Abrams, Burton. 'Long-term sleep apnea as a pathogenic factor for cell-mediated autoimmune disease.' *Med Hypotheses*. 2005; 65(6): 1024–27. doi: 10.1016/j.mehy.2005.05.046. Epub 2005 Aug 5. PMID:16084665.

[100] 'Study shows that people with sleep apnea have a high risk of death.' Press Release. AASM. August 1, 2008. https://aasm.org/study-shows-that-people-with-sleep-apnea-have-a-high-risk-of-death/.

[101] 'Circadian Rhythm Sleep Disorders: Diagnosis and Tests.' Cleveland Clinic. April 1, 2020. https://my.clevelandclinic.org/health/diseases/12115-circadian-rhythm-disorders/diagnosis-and-tests'

[102] Ibid.

[103] Ibid.

[104] Jamie Ducharme. 'People Are Sleeping in 20-Minute Bursts To Boost Productivity. But Is It Safe?' *Time*. Jan. 30, 2018. https://

time.com/5063665/what-is-polyphasic-sleep/.

[105] Circadian Rhythm Sleep Disorders. Cleveland Clinic.

[106] Dodson, Ehren R, and Phyllis C Zee. 'Therapeutics for Circadian Rhythm Sleep Disorders.' *Sleep Medicine Clinics* 5, 4 (2010): 701–15. doi:10.1016/j.jsmc.2010.08.001 https://www.ncbi.nlm.nih.gov/pmc/articles/PMC3020104/.

[107] Zhu, Lirong, and Phyllis C Zee. 'Circadian rhythm sleep disorders.' *Neurologic Clinics* 30, 4 (2012): 1167–91. doi:10.1016/j.ncl.2012.08.011. https://www.ncbi.nlm.nih.gov/pmc/articles/PMC3523094/.

[108] 'Narcolepsy, Definition.' Encyclopedia.com. https://www.encyclopedia.com/medicine/diseases-and-conditions/pathology/narcolepsy.

[109] 'Narcolepsy Fact Sheet.' NIH Neurological Institute. Mar 16, 2020. https://www.ninds.nih.gov/Disorders/Patient-Caregiver-Education/Fact-Sheets/Narcolepsy-Fact-Sheet.

[110] '9 Facts About Narcolepsy That May Surprise You.' *Narcolepsy, Sleep Disorder, Uncategorized.* Mar 2, 2016. https://valleysleepcenter.com/9-facts-about-narcolepsy-that-may-surprise-you/.

[111] Bonvalet, Melodie. 'Autoimmunity in narcolepsy.' *Curr Opin Pulm Med.* 2017 Nov; 23(6): 522–29. doi: 10.1097/MCP.0000000000000426. PMCID:PMC5773260.

[112] Mysliwiec, Vincent. 'Time for a standardized clinical assessment for narcolepsy with obstructive sleep apnea.' *Sleep Breath.* 2018 Mar; 22(1): 49–50. doi: 10.1007/s11325-017-1516-3. Epub 2017, Jun 16.

[113] Ohio State University. (2020, August 24). 'Each human gut has a viral 'fingerprint': New database consists of over 33,000 unique viral populations in the gut.' *ScienceDaily.* Retrieved September 25, 2020 from www.sciencedaily.com/releases/2020/08/200824131803.htm.

[114] Moossavi, Shirin, Arrieta, Marie-Claire. 'Gut reaction: How the gut microbiome may influence the severity of Covid-19.' *The Conversation.* June 21, 2020. https://theconversation.com/gut-reaction-how-the-gut-microbiome-may-influence-the-severity-of-covid-19-139094.

[115] Wang, Baohong, et al., 'The Human Microbiota in Health and Disease.' *Engineering.* Feb 2017; 3:1. 71–82. https://www.science-

direct.com/science/article/pii/S2095809917301492.

[116] Durack, Juliana. 'The gut microbiome: Relationships with disease and opportunities for therapy.' *J Exp Med.* 2019 Jan 7; 216(1): 20–40. doi: 10.1084/jem.20180448. Epub 2018 Oct 15. PMID: 30322864.

[117] Vieira, S. Manfredo. 'Translocation of a gut pathobiont drives autoimmunity in mice and humans.' *Science.* Mar 9, 2018; 359 (6380): 1156–61 DOI: 10.1126/science.aar7201.

[118] Balmer, Maria, et. al., 'The liver may act as a firewall mediating mutualism between the host and its gut commensal microbiota.' *Sci Transl Med.* 2014 May 21; 6(237): 237ra66. doi: 10.1126/scitranslmed.3008618. pmid:24848256.

[119] Wu Hsin-Jung. 'The role of gut microbiota in immune homeostasis and autoimmunity.' *Gut Microbes.* Jan-Feb 2012; 3(1): 4–14. doi: 10.4161/gmic.19320. Epub 2012, Jan 1. PMID: 22356853.

[120] Wang, Baohong, et al., 'The Human Microbiota in Health and Disease.' *Engineering.* Feb 2017; 3 (1): 71–82. https://www.sciencedirect.com/science/article/pii/S2095809917301492.

[121] Neuman, Hadar, et al., 'Antibiotics in early life: dysbiosis and the damage done.' *FEMS Microbiol Rev.* 2018 Jul 1; 42(4): 489–99. doi: 10.1093/femsre/fuy018.

[122] David, Lawrence A., et al., 'Gut Microbial Succession Follows Acute Secretory Diarrhea in Humans.' *American Society for Microbiology.* DOI: 10.1128/mBio.00381-15.

[123] Wang, Fuyuan, et al., 'Morphine induces changes in the gut microbiome and metabolome in a morphine dependence model.' *Sci Rep* 8, 3596 (2018). https://doi.org/10.1038/s41598-018-21915-8.

[124] 'Lead in U.S. Drinking Water.' *SciLine.* https://www.sciline.org/evidence-blog/lead-drinking-water.

[125] Samsel, Anthony. 'Glyphosate, pathways to modern diseases II: Celiac sprue and gluten intolerance.' *Interdiscip Toxicol.* 2013 Dec; 6(4): 159–84. doi: 10.2478/intox-2013-0026.

[126] Flannery, Jessica, et al., 'Gut Feelings Begin in Childhood: the Gut Metagenome Correlates with Early Environment, Caregiving, and Behavior.' *Clinical Science and Epidemiology, American Society for Microbiology.* Mar 12, 2019. DOI: 10.1128/mBio.02780-19.

[127] Kelly, John R, et al., 'Breaking down the barriers: the gut microbiome, intestinal permeability and stress-related psychiatric

disorders.' *Front. Cell. Neurosci.*, 14 October 2015. https://doi.org/10.3389/fncel.2015.00392.

[128] DuPont, Herbert, et al., 'Travel and travelers' diarrhea in patients with irritable bowel syndrome.' *Am J Trop Med Hyg.* 2010 Feb; 82(2): 301–5. doi: 10.4269/ajtmh.2010.09-0538.

[129] Das, P., et al. ,Metagenomic analysis of microbe-mediated vitamin metabolism in the human gut microbiome.' *BMC Genomics* 20, 208 (2019). https://doi.org/10.1186/s12864-019-5591-7.

[130] Rowland, Ian, et al., 'Gut microbiota functions: metabolism of nutrients and other food components.' *Eur J Nutr.* 2018 Feb; 57(1): 1–24. doi: 10.1007/s00394-017-1445-8. Epub 2017, Apr 9.

[131] 'Need More Magnesium? 10 Signs.' *EnviroMedica.* http://www.ancient-minerals.com/magnesium-deficiency/need-more/.

[132] Cohen, Suzy, R.Ph, '14 Drugs that Deplete Magnesium. Jigsaw Health.' *The Magnesium People.* Feb 3, 2015. http://www.jigsawhealth.com/blog/drug-muggers-suzy-cohen-magnesium.

[133] Patrick, Rhonda, Ph.D. 'Three Main Causes of Magnesium Deficiency (Part 2).' *Wellness FX.* http://blog.wellnessfx.com/2013/07/31/three-main-causes-of-magnesium-deficiency-part-2/; Jahnen-Dechent, W., Ketteler, M. ,Magnesium Basics.' *Clinical Kidney Journal* 5, 3–14 (210).

[134] Stern, Victoria. 'The Oxygen Dilemma: Can Too Much O2 Kill?' *Scientific American MIND.* Oct 1, 2008. https://www.scientificamerican.com/article/the-oxygen-dilemma/.

[135] Anderson, LV. 'The Kill of the Thrill.: Can you die from excitement?' *Slate.* July 9, 2012. http://www.slate.com/articles/health_and_science/explainer/2012/07/josephine_ann_harris_can_you_die_from_excitement.html.

[136] Ballantyne, Coco. 'Strange but True: Drinking Too Much Water Can Kill.' *Scientific American.* June 21, 2007. https://www.scientificamerican.com/article/strange-but-true-drinking-too-much-wat.

[137] Lawrence, Ph.D, Paige, et al., University of Rochester Medical Center. 'Environmental toxins impair immune system over multiple generations.' *ScienceDaily*, October 2, 2019. www.sciencedaily.com/releases/2019/10/191002144257.htm.

[138] Fasano A. Zonulin, 'Regulation of tight junctions, and autoimmune diseases.' *Ann N Y Acad Sci.* 2012; 1258(1): 25–33. doi:10.1111/j.1749-6632.2012.06538.x.

[139] 'Poisons and Toxins.' Science Learning Lab. https://www. sciencelearn.org.nz/resources/364-poisons-and-toxins.

[140] Household Products Database. U.S. Dept of Health & Human Services. https://hpd.nlm.nih.gov/cgi-bin/household/brands?tbl=chem&id=77.

[141] Leah Zerbe. 'Banish these 12 household toxins.' *Rodale Organic Life.* Jan 22, 2016. https://www.rodalesorganiclife.com/home/banish-these-12-household-toxins-from-your-house?slide=1/slide/8.

[142] 'Chapter 5: Indoor Air Pollutants and Toxic Materials.' Centers for Disease Control and Prevention and U.S. Department of Housing and Urban Development. *Healthy Housing Reference Manual.* Atlanta: US Department of Health and Human Services; 2006. https://www.cdc.gov/nceh/publications/books/housing/cha05.htm.

[143] 'Fact Sheet: Octane.' Environmental and Energy Study Institute EESI. March 2016. https://www.eesi.org/files/FactSheet_Octane_History_2016.pdf.

[144] 'More than 4 in 10 Americans Live with Unhealthy Air; Eight Cities Suffered Most Polluted Air Ever Recorded.' American Lung Association. Apr 24, 2019. https://www.lung.org/media/press-releases/sota-2019.

[145] McNulty, Jennier. 'Coastal fog linked to high levels of mercury found in mountain lions, study finds.' *UCSC.* Nov 26, 2019. https://news.ucsc.edu/2019/11/wilmers-mercury.html.

[146] Levesque, Shannon, et al., 'Air pollution & the brain: Subchronic diesel exhaust exposure causes neuroinflammation and elevates early markers of neurodegenerative disease.' *J Neuroinflammation* 8, 105 (2011). https://doi.org/10.1186/1742-2094-8-105 https://link.springer.com/article/10.1186/1742-2094-8-105.

[147] Fact Sheet: Octane.

[148] Fact Sheet: Octane.

[149] Michael McCarthy. 'Lead-free petrol may be villain in mystery of demise of the world's most familiar bird.' *The Independent.* Sept 11, 2000. https://www.independent.co.uk/environment/lead-free-petrol-may-be-villain-in-mystery-of-demise-of-the-worlds-most-familiar-bird-698469.html.

[150] 'Fact Sheet: Octane.' Environmental and Energy Study Institute EESI. March 2016. https://www.eesi.org/files/FactSheet_Octane_History_2016.pdf.

[151] Libby Longino. 'Researchers stumped over decline of sparrow population.' *USA Today.* Oct 5, 2013. https://eu.usatoday.com/story/news/world/2013/10/05/sparrows-dying/2923241/.

[152] McCarthy. Ibid.

[153] Ibid.

[154] Heid, Markham. 'How to Avoid Vehicle Pollution When You're Stuck in Traffic.' *Time.* Aug 19, 2019. https://time.com/5655400/traffic-air-pollution/.

[155] Ibid.

[156] 'Drinking Water.' EPA https://www.epa.gov/report-environment/drinking-water.

[157] Rhea Suh. 'We can't assume our water is safe to drink. But we can fix it.' *National Geographic.* March 2019. https://www.nationalgeographic.com/magazine/2019/03/drinking-water-safety-in-united-sates-can-be-fixed/.

[158] Ibid.

[159] Melissa Young, MD. 'Environmental Toxins and Your Health.' Cleveland Clinic online health chat. June 3, 2014. https://my.clevelandclinic.org/health/transcripts/1622_environmental-toxins-and-your-health.

[160] 'Consumer Reports. You're literally eating microplastics. How you can cut down exposure to them.' *The Washington Post.* Oct 7 2019. https://www.washingtonpost.com/health/youre-literally-eating-microplastics-how-you-can-cut-down-exposure-to-them/2019/10/04/22ebdfb6-e17a-11e9-8dc8-498eabc129a0_story.html.

[161] Heid, Markham. How to Avoid Vehicle Pollution.

[162] 'Mold Pollution.' *Pollution Issues.* http://www.pollutionissues.com/Li-Na/Mold-Pollution.html.

[163] Mudarri, David H. 'Valuing the Economic Costs of Allergic Rhinitis, Acute Bronchitis, and Asthma from Exposure to Indoor Dampness and Mold in the US.' *Journal of Environmental and Public Health.* May 29, 2016; 2016, Article ID 2386596, http://dx.doi.org/10.1155/2016/2386596.

[164] Tuuminen, Tamara, et al., 'Severe Sequelae to Mold-Related Illness as Demonstrated in Two Finnish Cohorts.' *Front. Immunol.,* Apr 3, 2017. https://doi.org/10.3389/fimmu.2017.00382.

[165] 'Prevalence of Building Dampness. Scientific Findings Re-

source Bank.' Indoor Air Quality. https://iaqscience.lbl.gov/damp-ness-prevalence.

[166] Franklin, Delano R., et al. 'Mold Plagues "Virtually All Build-ings," Dean Says After Dunster Mold Outbreak. *Harvard Crimson*. Nov 8, 2019. https://www.thecrimson.com/article/2019/11/8/dun-ster-mold-outbreak/.

[167] 'Everything You Need To Know About Environmental Toxins And Their Effects On Your Health.' *Quicksilver Scientific*. Feb 7, 2020. https://www.quicksilverscientific.com/blog/everything-you-need-to-know-about-environmental-toxins-and-their-effects-on-your-health/.

[168] Amy Waterman. 'Heavy Metal Toxicity & Contamination: What You Need To Know.' *Hydroviv*. June 28, 2017.

[169] Ibid.

[170] Ibid.

[171] Ibid.

[172] Mary Jane Brown, PhD. 'Should You Avoid Fish Because of Mercury?' *Healthline*. Sept 14, 2016. https://www.healthline.com/nutrition/mercury-content-of-fish?utm_medium=email&utm_source=email-share&utm_campaign=social-sharebar-re-ferred-desktop.

[173] 'Choose the Right Fish To Lower Mercury Risk Exposure.' *Consumer Reports*. May 4, 2019. https://www.consumerreports.org/cro/magazine/2014/10/can-eating-the-wrong-fish-put-you-at-higher-risk-for-mercury-exposure/index.htm.

[174] Ibid.

[175] Ibid.

[176] Mary Jane Brown, PhD. 'Should You Avoid Fish Because of Mercury?' *Healthline*. Sept 14, 2016. https://www.healthline.com/nutrition/mercury-content-of-fish?utm_medium=email&utm_source=email-share&utm_campaign=social-sharebar-re-ferred-desktop.

[177] Carey Gillam. 'Weedkiller products more toxic than their active ingredient, tests show.' *The Guardian*. May 8, 2018. https://www.theguardian.com/us-news/2018/may/08/weedkiller-tests-monsan-to-health-dangers-active-ingredient.

[178] Ibid.

[179] Ibid.

[180] Ibid.

[181] Ibid.

[182] 'What's The Connection Between Glyphosate And Genetically Modified Crops?' *The Detox Project*. https://detoxproject.org/glyphosate/whats-the-connection-between-glyphosate-and-genetically-modified-crops/.

[183] Samsel, Anthony. 'Glyphosate, pathways to modern diseases.'

[184] Parks, Christine G., et al., 'Insecticide Use And Risk Of Rheumatoid Arthritis And Systemic Lupus Erythematosus In The Women's Health Initiative Observational Study.' *Arthritis Care Res* (Hoboken). 2011 Feb; 63(2): 184–94. doi: 10.1002/acr.20335 PMC3593584.

[185] 'Glyphosate Toxicity. Functional Wisdom...healthy updates from Dr. Barbara!' Nov 24, 2015. https://doccarnahan.blogspot.com/.

[186] 'Trauma. Early Childhood Mental Health.' Missouri Department of Mental Health. https://dmh.mo.gov/healthykids/providers/trauma.

[187] Song H, Fall K, Fang F, et al. ,Stress related disorders and subsequent risk of life threatening infections: population based sibling controlled cohort study.' *BMJ*. 2019, Oct 23; 367: l5784. doi:10.1136/bmj.l5784.

[188] Ibid.

[189] Song H, Sieurin J, Wirdefeldt K, et al. 'Association of Stress-Related Disorders With Subsequent Neurodegenerative Diseases.' *JAMA Neurol*. 2020; 77(6): 1–11. doi:10.1001/jamaneurol.2020.0117.

[190] 'Trauma.' American Psychological Association. https://www.apa.org/topics/trauma#:~:text=Trauma%20is%20an%20emotional%20response,symptoms%20like%20headaches%20or%20nausea.

[191] Susanne Babbel MFT, PhD. 'The Trauma That Arises from Natural Disasters.' *Psychology Today*. Apr 21, 2010. https://www.psychologytoday.com/us/blog/somatic-psychology/201004/the-trauma-arises-natural-disasters.

[192] Robert H. Shmerling, MD. 'Autoimmune disease and stress: Is there a link?' Harvard Medical School. July 11, 2018. https://www.health.harvard.edu/blog/autoimmune-disease-and-stress-is-there-a-link-2018071114230.

[193] 'How to Cope with Traumatic Events like Coronavirus.' *Help*

Guide. https://www.helpguide.org/articles/ptsd-trauma/traumatic-stress.htm.

[194] 'Trauma. Early Childhood Mental Health.' Missouri Department of Mental Health. https://dmh.mo.gov/healthykids/providers/trauma.

[195] Ibid.

[196] Virginia Hughes. 'The Roots of Resilience.' *Nature.* 2012, Oct 11; 490: 165–167.

[197] Robert H. Shmerling, MD. 'Autoimmune disease and stress: Is there a link?' Harvard Medical School. July 11, 2018. https://www.health.harvard.edu/blog/autoimmune-disease-and-stress-is-there-a-link-2018071114230.

[198] Virginia Hughes. The Roots of Resilience.

[199] Song H, Fang F, Tomasson G, et al. 'Association of Stress-Related Disorders With Subsequent Autoimmune Disease.' *JAMA.* 2018; 319(23): 2388–2400. doi:10.1001/jama.2018.7028.

[200] Ibid.

[201] 'Trauma. Early Childhood Mental Health.'

[202] 'Toxic Stress. Center for the Developing Child.' Harvard University. https://developingchild.harvard.edu/science/key-concepts/toxic-stress/

[203] 'Trauma. Early Childhood Mental Health.'

[204] 'Preventing Adverse Childhood Experiences. Violence Prevention.' Centers for Disease Control. https://www.cdc.gov/violenceprevention/childabuseandneglect/aces/fastfact.html.

[205] Ibid.

[206] Ibid.

[207] Ibid.

[208] 'About the CDC-Kaiser ACE Study. Violence Prevention.' Centers for Disease Control. https://www.cdc.gov/violenceprevention/childabuseandneglect/acestudy/about.html.

[209] Vincent J Felitti MD, FACP, et al., 'Relationship of Childhood Abuse and Household Dysfunction to Many of the Leading Causes of Death in Adults: The Adverse Childhood Experiences (ACE) Study.' DOI: https://doi.org/10.1016/S0749-3797(98)00017-8 https://www.ajpmonline.org/article/S0749-3797(98)00017-8/abstract.

[210] Ibid.

[211] 'We Protect Children from ACEs.' Stop Abuse Campaign. https://stopabusecampaign.org/

[212] Ibid.

[213] Ibid.

[214] 'Memories of Childhood Abuse.' American Psychological Association. https://www.apa.org/topics/trauma/memories

[215] Ibid.

[216] Garvey MA, Giedd J, Swedo SE. 'PANDAS: the search for environmental triggers of pediatric neuropsychiatric disorders. Lessons from rheumatic fever.' *Journal of Child Neurology*. Sept 1998;13(9): 413–23. DOI: 10.1177/088307389801300901.

[217] Swedo, SE, et al., 'From Research Subgroup to Clinical Syndrome: Modifying the PANDAS Criteria to Describe PANS. Pediatric Acute-onset Neuropsychiatric Syndrome.' *Pediatr Therapeut* 2012, 2: 2. DOI: 10.4172/2161-0665.1000113.

[218] Ercan TE, Ercan G, Severge B, Arpaozu M, Karasu G. 'Mycoplasma pneumoniae infection and obsessive-compulsive disease: a case report.' *Journal of Child Neurology*. 2008 Mar; 23(3): 338–40. DOI: 10.1177/0883073807308714.

[219] 'Ehlers-Danlos syndrome. Genetics Home Reference.' *Medline Plus*. https://medlineplus.gov/genetics/condition/ehlers-danlos-syndrome/#diagnosis.

[220] 'EDS Types.' The Ehlers-Danlos Society. https://www.ehlers-danlos.com/eds-types/#cEDS.

[221] Kiesel, Laura. 'Ehlers-Danlos Syndrome.' *Harvard Health Publishing*. Harvard Medical School. Aug 7, 2017. https://www.health.harvard.edu/blog/ehlers-danlos-syndrome-mystery-solved-2017080712122.

[222] Scheper MC, de Vries JE, Verbunt J, Engelbert RH. 'Chronic pain in hypermobility syndrome and Ehlers-Danlos syndrome (hypermobility type): it is a challenge.' *Journal of Pain Research*. 2015; 8: 591–601. DOI: 10.2147/jpr.s64251.

[223] Kiesel, L. 'Ehlers-Danlos syndrome: A mystery solved.' *Harvard Medical School Publishing*. Aug 7, 2017. https://www.health.harvard.edu/blog/ehlers-danlos-syndrome-mystery-solved-2017080712122.

[224] Roma, M. et al., 'Postural tachycardia syndrome and other forms of orthostatic intolerance in Ehlers-Danlos syndrome.' *Autonomic Neuroscience Review*. 2018, Dec 1; 215, 89–96, https://doi.org/10.1016/j.autneu.2018.02.006.

[225] Marques A. 'Chronic Lyme disease: a review.' Infectious Dis-

ease Clinics of North America. 2008 Jun; 22(2): 341–60, vii-viii. DOI: 10.1016/j.idc.2007.12.011.PMID: 18452806.

[226] Ibid.

[227] Waddell LA, Greig J, Mascarenhas M, et al. 'The Accuracy of Diagnostic Tests for Lyme Disease in Humans, A Systematic Review and Meta-Analysis of North American Research.' *Plos One.* 2016; 11(12): e0168613. DOI: 10.1371/journal.pone.0168613.

[228] Pachner, AR. 'Neurologic manifestations of Lyme disease, the new "great imitator."' *Rev Infect Dis.* Sep–Oct 1989; 11 Suppl 6: S1482–6. PMID: 2682960.

[229] Moutailler S, Valiente Moro C, Vaumourin E, et al. 'Co-infection of Ticks: The Rule Rather Than the Exception.' *Plos Neglected Tropical Diseases.* 2016 Mar; 10(3): e0004539. DOI: 10.1371/journal.pntd.0004539. PMID: 26986203.

[230] Eisen, RJ, et al., 'The Blacklegged Tick, Ixodes scapularis: An Increasing Public Health Concern.' *Trends Parasitol.* 2018 Apr; 34(4): 295–309. PMCID: PMC5879012.

[231] Bernard, Q. et al., 'Plasticity in early immune evasion strategies of a bacterial pathogen.' *Proc Natl Acad Sci U S A.* 2018, Apr 17; 115(16): E3788-E3797. doi: 10.1073/pnas.1718595115. Epub 2018 Apr 2. PMID: 29610317.

[232] Horowitz RI, Freeman PR. 'Precision medicine: retrospective chart review and data analysis of 200 patients on dapsone combination therapy for chronic Lyme disease/post-treatment Lyme disease syndrome: part 1.' *International Journal of General Medicine.* 2019; 12:101–19. DOI: 10.2147/ijgm.s193608.

[233] Cahalan, S. *Brain on Fire: My Month of Madness* (New York: Simon & Schuster, 2012).

[234] 'Lyme disease—Reported cases* by year, United States, 1997-2017. Lyme Disease Charts and Figures: Historical Data.' Centers for Disease Control and Prevention. https://www.cdc.gov/lyme/stats/graphs.html.

[235] Morris G, Berk M, Maes M, Carvalho AF, Puri BK. 'Socioeconomic Deprivation, Adverse Childhood Experiences and Medical Disorders in Adulthood: Mechanisms and Associations.' *Molecular Neurobiology.* 2019 Aug; 56(8): 5866–90. DOI: 10.1007/s12035-019-1498-1. PMID: 30685844.

[236] Dantzer R, Cohen S, Russo SJ, Dinan TG. 'Resilience and

immunity.' *Brain, Behavior, and Immunity*. 2018 Nov; 74: 28–42. DOI: 10.1016/j.bbi.2018.08.010. PMID: PMC30102966

[237] Ibid.

[238] Black DS, Slavich GM. 'Mindfulness meditation and the immune system: a systematic review of randomized controlled trials.' *Annals of the New York Academy of Sciences*. 2016 Jun; 1373(1): 13–24. DOI: 10.1111/nyas.12998.PMID: 26799456.

[239] 'Lyme Disease.' Centers for Disease Control and Prevention. https://www.cdc.gov/lyme/index.html.

[240] 'Borrelia burgdorferi. ScienceDirect. from David H. Spach.' *The Travel and Tropical Medicine Manual*. (4th ed. Elsevier, 2008) ed. Elaine C. Jong and Christopher Sanford. Ch. 23

[241] Hu, Linden MD. 'Patient education: Lyme disease symptoms and diagnosis' (Beyond the Basics). Up to Date. https://www.uptodate.com/contents/lyme-disease-symptoms-and-diagnosis-beyond-the-basics.

[242] 'What to be Tested For.' *Global Lyme Alliance*. https://globallymealliance.org/about-lyme/diagnosis/testing.

[243] 'Your Lyme Disease Test Results Are Negative, But Your Symptoms Say Otherwise.' *IGenex*. https://igenex.com/tick-talk/your-lyme-disease-test-results-are-negative-but-your-symptoms-say-otherwise/.

[244] Caruso, Catherine. 'Tests for Lyme disease miss many early cases — but a new approach could help.' *Stat*. June 28, 2017. https://www.statnews.com/2017/06/28/early-lyme-tests/.

[245] Stone, Judy. 'The Lyme Wars: Major Organizations Aren't Playing Nicely Together.' *Forbes*. Aug 2, 2019. https://www.forbes.com/sites/judystone/2019/08/02/the-lyme-wars-major-organizations-arent-playing-nicely-together/#6695f97243c4.

[246] Specter, Michael. 'The Lyme Wars'. *The New Yorker*. June 24, 2013. https://www.newyorker.com/magazine/2013/07/01/the-lyme-wars.

[247] Shor S, Green C, Szantyr B, et al. 'Chronic Lyme Disease: An Evidence-Based Definition by the ILADS Working Group.' *Antibiotics (Basel)*. 2019, Dec 16; 8(4): 269.doi:10.3390/antibiotics8040269.

[248] Citera M, Freeman PR, Horowitz RI. 'Empirical validation of the Horowitz Multiple Systemic Infectious Disease Syndrome

Questionnaire for suspected Lyme disease.' *Int J Gen Med.* 2017, Sep 4;10: 249–73.doi:10.2147/IJGM.S140224.

[249] Maggi, Ricardo. 'In Pursuit of a Stealth Pathogen: Laboratory Diagnosis of Bartonellosis.' *Clinical Microbiology Newsletter,* 2014. https://www.academia.edu/33554781/In_Pursuit_of_a_Stealth_Pathogen_Laboratory_Diagnosis_of_Bartonellosis.

[250] *Innate Immunity and Inflammation.* Ruslan M. Medzhitov, ed. Yale University School of Medicine, 2015. https://cshperspectives. cshlp.org/site/misc/innate_immunity_and_inflammation.xhtml.

[251] Albrecht, Daniel, et al., 'Brain glial activation in fibromyalgia – A multi-site positron emission tomography investigation.' *Brain, Behavior, and Immunity.* Jan 2019; 75: 72–83. doi: 10.1016/j. bbi.2018.09.018; Nordengen, Kaja. 'Glial activation and inflammation along the Alzheimer's disease continuum.' *Journal of Neuroinflammation.* Feb 21, 2019. doi.org/10.1186/s12974-019-1399-2.

[252] 'Mast Cell. Biology.' *Britannica.* https://www.britannica.com/ science/mast-cell.

[253] Moyer, Nancy. Elaine K. Luo, MD. 'Mast Cell Activation Syndrome.' *Healthline.* May 30, 2019. https://www.healthline.com/ health/mast-cell-activation-syndrome.

[254] Rogers, Kara. 'Microglia.' *Britannica.* https://www.britannica. com/science/microglia.

[255] The Cunningham Panel. Moleculera Labs Educational Series. https://www.moleculeralabs.com/cunningham-pan- el-results-help-determine-treatment-plan-child-schizophren- ic-like-symptoms/

[256] Ibid.

[257] Ibid.

Shimasaki, Craig, et al. 'Evaluation of the Cunningham Panel™ in pediatric autoimmune neuropsychiatric disorder associated with streptococcal infection (PANDAS) and pediatric acute-onset neuropsychiatric syndrome (PANS): Changes in antineuronal antibody titers parallel changes in patient symptoms.' *Journal of Neuroimmunology.* 2020, Feb 15; 339, 577138. https://doi.org/10.1016/j.jneuroim.2019.577138.

[258] The Cunningham Panel. PANS / PANDAS. https://aonm.org/ cunningham-panel-panspandas/

[259] Ibid.

[260] ADRESS LATER 3 different citations numbered 5

[261] 'Can people with type 2 diabetes stop taking metformin?' *MedicalNewsToday*. https://www.medicalnewstoday.com/articles/323128.

[262] Ursini, Francesco. 'Metformin and Autoimmunity: A "New Deal" of an Old Drug.' *Front. Immunol.*, June 4, 2018. https://doi.org/10.3389/fimmu.2018.01236.

[263] Sharma S, Ray A, Sadasivam B. 'Metformin in Covid-19: A possible role beyond diabetes.' *Diabetes Res Clin Pract.* 2020;164:108183. doi:10.1016/j.diabres.2020.108183.

[264] Grattendick, Kenneth. Susan Pross. Immunoglobulins in xPharm: The Comprehensive Pharmacology Reference, eds. S.J. Enna and David B. Bylund. (Elsevier, 2008). https://www.sciencedirect.com/topics/neuroscience/intravenous-immunoglobulin

[265] 'Intravenous Immunoglobulin Therapy (IVIg).' *WebMD*. https://www.webmd.com/a-to-z-guides/immunoglobulin-therapy#1.

[266] 'Plasmapheresis: Side effects and how it works.' *MedicalNewsToday*. https://www.medicalnewstoday.com/articles/321451.

[267] McGinley, Marisa P., Brandon P. Moss & Jeffrey A. Cohen, 'Safety of monoclonal antibodies for the treatment of multiple sclerosis.' *Expert Opinion on Drug Safety*. 2017; 16: 1, 89–100, DOI: 10.1080/14740338.2017.1250881.

[268] Maria Paul. 'Popular Cancer Drug Linked To Often Fatal "Brain Eating" Virus.' *Northwester*. May 20, 2009. https://www.northwestern.edu/newscenter/stories/2009/05/bennett.html.

[269] Clinical Management of Pediatric Acute-Onset Neuropsychiatric Syndrome: Part III—Treatment and Prevention of Infections, Michael S. Cooperstock, Susan E. Swedo, Mark S. Pasternack, Tanya K. Murphy, 'The PANS/PANDAS Consortium.' *Journal of Child and Adolescent Psychopharmacology* 2017; 27: 7, 594–606.

[270] https://www.fiercebiotech.com/research/stem-cells-don-t-repair-injured-hearts-but-inflammation-might-study-finds86

[271] 'Stem Cell Therapy for Autoimmune Diseases.' Stem Cell Institute. https://www.cellmedicine.com/stem-cell-therapy-for-autoimmune-diseases/

[272] Ibid.

[273] 'Chapter 6: Autoimmune Diseases and the Promise of Stem Cell-Based Therapies. Stem Cells: Scientific Progress and Future

Research Directions.' National Institutes of Health. U.S. Department of Health and Human Services. June 17, 2001. https://stemcells.nih.gov/info/2001report/chapter6.htm.

[274] Hui Xu, Shaochang Jia, Hanmei Xu. 'Potential therapeutic applications of exosomes in different autoimmune diseases.' *Clinical Immunology* August 2019; 205: 116–24. https://www.sciencedirect.com/science/article/abs/pii/S1521661619301548.

[275] 'FDA Warns About Stem Cell Therapies.' U.S. Food & Drug Administration. https://www.fda.gov/consumers/consumer-updates/fda-warns-about-stem-cell-therapies.

[276] Thomas M. Heffron. 'Sleep and Caffeine.' *SleepEducation. org*, Aug 1, 2013. http://sleepeducation.org/news/2013/08/01/sleep-and-caffeine#:~:text=The%20most%20obvious%20effect%20of,deep%20sleep%20that%20you%20enjoy.

[277] Ates, Mehmet, et al., 'Dose-Dependent Absorption Profile of Different Magnesium Compounds.' *Biol Trace Elem Res.* Dec 2019; 192(2): 244–51. doi: 10.1007/s12011-019-01663-0. Epub 2019 Feb 13.PMID:30761462.

[278] Mayo Clinic Staff. 'Insomnia treatment: Cognitive behavioral therapy instead of sleeping pills.' Mayo Clinic. https://www.mayoclinic.org/diseases-conditions/insomnia/in-depth/insomnia-treatment/art-20046677.

[279] Ibid.

[280] Ostrin, Lisa A., et al. 'Attenuation of short wavelengths alters sleep and the ipRGC pupil response.' *OPO.* July 2017; 37: 4, 440–50. June 27, 2017. https://doi.org/10.1111/opo.12385.

[281] Shergis, JL, et al. 'A systematic review of acupuncture for sleep quality in people with insomnia.' *Complementary Therapies in Medicine.* June 2016; 26: 11–20. https://doi.org/10.1016/j.ctim.2016.02.007.

[282] He, Wenbo, et. al., 'Acupuncture for treatment of insomnia: An overview of systematic reviews.' *Complementary Therapies in Medicine.* Feb 2019; 42: 407–16. https://doi.org/10.1016/j.ctim.2018.12.020.

[283] Ong, JC., et. al, 'A randomized controlled trial of mindfulness meditation for chronic insomnia.' *Sleep.* 2014, Sep 1; 37(9): 1553–63. doi: 10.5665/sleep.4010.

[284] 'Diagnosis. Sleep apnea.' Mayo Clinic. https://www.mayoclinic.org/diseases-conditions/sleep-apnea/diagnosis-treatment/drc-20377636.

[285] 'Top 5 Reasons People Quit Using the CPAP.' *Cure My Sleep Apnea.* May 13, 2015. http://curemysleepapnea.com/sleep-source/2015/05/13/top-5-reasons-people-quit-using-cpap/.

[286] 'Sleep Apnea Treatment Options.' American Sleep Apnea Association https://www.sleepapnea.org/treat/sleep-apnea-treatment-options/.

[287] Logsdon AF, Erickson MA, Rhea EM, Salameh TS, Banks WA. ,Gut reactions: How the blood-brain barrier connects the microbiome and the brain.' *Exp Biol Med (Maywood).* 2018; 243(2): 159–65. doi:10.1177/1535370217743766.

[288] Vighi G, Marcucci F, Sensi L, Di Cara G, Frati F. 'Allergy and the gastrointestinal system.' *Clin Exp Immunol.* 2008; 153 (Suppl 1): 3–6. doi:10.1111/j.1365-2249.2008.03713.

[289] Bouzia, Romain, et al., 'Reovirus infection triggers inflammatory responses to dietary antigens and development of celiac disease.' *Science*, 2017, 7 Apr; 356 (6333): 44–50. DOI: 10.1126/science.aah5298.

[290] 'Celiac Disease Facts and Figures.' Celiac Disease Center. University of Chicago School of Medicine. https://www.cureceliacdisease.org/wp-content/uploads/341_CDCFactSheets8_FactsFigures.pdf.

[291] Fedewa A, Rao SS. 'Dietary fructose intolerance, fructan intolerance and FODMAPs.' *Curr Gastroenterol Rep.* 2014; 16(1): 370. doi:10.1007/s11894-013-0370-0.

[292] Mindikoglu, Ayse L., et. al., 'Intermittent fasting from dawn to sunset for 30 consecutive days is associated with anticancer proteomic signature and upregulates key regulatory proteins of glucose and lipid metabolism, circadian clock, DNA repair, cytoskeleton remodeling, immune system and cognitive function in healthy subjects.' *Journal of Proteomics.* April 15, 2020; 217: 103645. https://doi.org/10.1016/j.jprot.2020.103645.

[293] 'Chapter 5: Indoor Air Pollutants and Toxic Materials.' Centers for Disease Control and Prevention and U.S. Department of Housing and Urban Development. Healthy housing reference manual. Atlanta: US Department of Health and Human Services; 2006. https://www.cdc.gov/nceh/publications/books/housing/cha05.htm.

[294] Davani-Davari D, Negahdaripour M, Karimzadeh I, et al. 'Prebiotics: Definition, Types, Sources, Mechanisms, and Clinical Applications.' *Foods.* 2019, Mar 9; 8(3): 92. doi:10.3390/foods8030092.

[295] Basaranoglu M, Basaranoglu G, Sabuncu T, Sentürk H. 'Fructose as a key player in the development of fatty liver disease.' *World J Gastroenterol.* 2013; 19(8): 1166–72. doi:10.3748/wjg.v19.i8.1166.

[296] Softic S, Cohen DE, Kahn CR. 'Role of Dietary Fructose and Hepatic De Novo Lipogenesis in Fatty Liver Disease.' *Dig Dis Sci.* 2016; 61(5): 1282–93. doi:10.1007/s10620-016-4054-0.

[297] Navarro, Victor J et al. 'Liver injury from herbal and dietary supplements.' *Hepatology* (Baltimore, Md.). 2017; 65 (1): 363–73. doi:10.1002/hep.28813

[298] Roytman, M. M., Poerzgen, P., & Navarro, V. (2018). 'Botanicals and hepatotoxicity.' *Clinical Pharmacology & Therapeutics* 104 (3), 458–69.

[299] Abenavoli L, Capasso R, Milic N, Capasso F. 'Milk thistle in liver diseases: past, present, future.' *Phytother Res.* 2010; 24(10): 1423–32. doi:10.1002/ptr.3207.

[300] Abenavoli L, Izzo AA, Milić N, Cicala C, Santini A, Capasso R. 'Milk thistle (Silybum marianum): A concise overview on its chemistry, pharmacological, and nutraceutical uses in liver diseases.' *Phytother Res.* 2018; 32(11): 2202–13. doi:10.1002/ptr.6171.

[301] ???

[302] Nagashimada M, Ota T. 'Role of vitamin E in nonalcoholic fatty liver disease.' *IUBMB Life.* 2019; 71(4): 516–22. doi:10.1002/iub.1991.

[303] González-Castejón M, Visioli F, Rodriguez-Casado A. 'Diverse biological activities of dandelion.' *Nutr Rev.* 2012; 70(9): 534–47. doi:10.1111/j.1753-4887.2012.00509.

[304] Birben E, Sahiner UM, Sackesen C, Erzurum S, Kalayci O. ‚Oxidative stress and antioxidant defense.' *World Allergy Organ J.* 2012; 5(1): 9–19. doi:10.1097/WOX.0b013e3182439613.

[305] Silverman MN, Deuster PA. ‚Biological mechanisms underlying the role of physical fitness in health and resilience.' *Interface Focus.* 2014; 4(5): 20140040. doi:10.1098/rsfs.2014.0040.

[306] Mee-Inta O, Zhao ZW, Kuo YM. 'Physical Exercise Inhibits Inflammation and Microglial Activation.' *Cells.* 2019; 8(7): 691. Published Jul 9, 2019. doi:10.3390/cells8070691.

[307] Birben E, Sahiner UM, et al., 'Oxidative stress and antioxidant defense.' *World Allergy Organ J.* 2012; 5(1): 9–19. doi:10.1097/WOX.0b013e3182439613.

[308] Martens CR, Denman BA, Mazzo MR, et al. 'Chronic nicotinamide riboside supplementation is well-tolerated and elevates NAD+ in healthy middle-aged and older adults.' *Nat Commun.* 2018; 9(1): 1286. Published Mar 29, 2018. doi:10.1038/s41467-018-03421-7.

[309] Brewer JH, Thrasher JD, Hooper D. 'Chronic illness associated with mold and mycotoxins: is naso-sinus fungal biofilm the culprit?' *Toxins (Basel).* 2013; 6(1): 66–80. Published Dec 24, 2013. doi:10.3390/toxins6010066.

[310] Brewer JH, Thrasher JD, Hooper D. 'Chronic illness associated with mold and mycotoxins: is naso-sinus fungal biofilm the culprit?' *Toxins (Basel).* 2013, Dec 24; 6(1): 66–80.doi:10.3390/toxins6010066.

[311] Amy Waterman. 'Heavy Metal Toxicity & Contamination: What You Need To Know.' *Hydroviv.* June 28, 2017.

[312] Ibid.

[313] Mary Jane Brown, PhD. 'Should You Avoid Fish Because of Mercury?' *Healthline.* Sept 14, 2016. https://www.healthline.com/nutrition/mercury-content-of-fish?utm_medium=email&utm_source=email-share&utm_campaign=social-sharebar-referred-desktop.

[314] Ibid.

[315] Tang G, Tu X, Feng P. 'Lead Poisoning Caused by Traditional Chinese Medicine: A Case Report and Literature Review.' *Tohoku J Exp Med.* 2017; 243(2): 127–31. doi:10.1620/tjem.243.127.

[316] Marek A. Mikulski, Michael D. Wichman, Donald L. Simmons, Anthony N. Pham, Valentina Clottey & Laurence J. Fuortes, 'Toxic metals in ayurvedic preparations from a public health lead poisoning cluster investigation, International Journal of Occupational and Environmental Health.' 2017; 23 (3): 187–92, DOI: 10.1080/10773525.2018.1447880.

[317] Shaw, Hank. 'Mercury Levels in Fish.' Dec 6, 2019. https://www.thespruceeats.com/check-fish-for-mercury-before-buying-1300629.

[318] Bernhoft RA. 'Mercury toxicity and treatment: a review of the literature.' *J Environ Public Health.* 2012; 460508. doi:10.1155/2012/460508.

[319] Ibid.

[320] Sears ME. 'Chelation: harnessing and enhancing heavy metal

detoxification—a review.' *ScientificWorldJournal*. 2013, Apr 18; 219840., 2013. doi:10.1155/2013/219840.

[321] Amadi, C.N., Offor, S.J., Frazzoli, C. et al. 'Natural antidotes and management of metal toxicity.' 2019. *Environ Sci Pollut Res* 26, 18032–18052. https://doi.org/10.1007/s11356-019-05104-2.

[322] Merchant RE, Andre CA. 'A review of recent clinical trials of the nutritional supplement Chlorella pyrenoidosa in the treatment of fibromyalgia, hypertension, and ulcerative colitis.' *Altern Ther Health Med*. 2001; 7(3): 79–91.

[323] Panahi Y, Darvishi B, Jowzi N, Beiraghdar F, Sahebkar A. 'Chlorella vulgaris: A Multifunctional Dietary Supplement with Diverse Medicinal Properties.' *Curr Pharm Des*. 2016; 22(2): 164–73. doi:10.2174/1381612822666151112145226.

[324] Carey Gillam. 'Weedkiller products more toxic than their active ingredient, tests show.' *The Guardian*. May 8, 2018. https://www. theguardian.com/us-news/2018/may/08/weedkiller-tests-monsan-to-health-dangers-active-ingredient.

[325] Rueda-Ruzafa L, Cruz F, Roman P, Cardona D. 'Gut microbiota and neurological effects of glyphosate.' *Neurotoxicology*. 2019; 75: 1–8. doi:10.1016/j.neuro.2019.08.006.

[326] 'IARC Monographs Volume 112: evaluation of five organophosphate insecticides and herbicides.' International Agency for Research on Cancer, World Health Organization. Mar 20, 2015. https://www.iarc.fr/wp-content/uploads/2018/07/MonographVolume112-1.pdf.

[327] 'About Us.' The Environmental Working Group. https://www. ewg.org/about-us.

[328] Pizzorno J. 'Conventional Laboratory Tests to Assess Toxin Burden.' *Integr Med (Encinitas)*. 2015; 14(5): 8–16.

[329] Bonnie Bright, PhD. 'Trauma and the Soul: Psychoanalytic Approaches to the Inner World An Interview with Jungian Analyst Donald Kalsched.' *Pacifica Post*. Pacifica Graduate Institute. May 23, 2017. https://www.pacificapost.com/trauma-and-the-soul-psy-choanalytic-approaches-to-the-inner-world.

[330] 'Common Responses to Trauma and Coping Strategies.' Resources. Trauma Center. http://www.traumacenter.org/resources/tc_resources.php.

[331] Ibid.

[332] Bonnie Bright, PhD. Trauma and the Soul: Psychoanalytic

Approaches to the Inner World An Interview with Jungian Analyst Donald Kalsched. Pacifica Post. Pacifica Graduate Institute. May 23, 2017. https://www.pacificapost.com/trauma-and-the-soul-psychoanalytic-approaches-to-the-inner-world

[333] Ronald K. Siegel, Ph.D. *Intoxication: The Universal Drive for Mind-Altering Substances* (Park Street Press, 2005) third edition, https://www.amazon.com/Intoxication-Universal-Drive-Mind-Altering-Substances/dp/1594770697/ref=sr_1_1?dchild=1&keywords=intoxication&qid=1592093338&s=books&sr=1-1.

[334] Huan Song, MD, PhD; Fang Fang, MD, PhD, et al. ,Association of Stress-Related Disorders With Subsequent Autoimmune Disease.' *JAMA*. 2018; 319(23): 2388–2400. doi:10.1001/jama.2018.7028.

[335] Sareen J. 'Posttraumatic stress disorder in adults: impact, comorbidity, risk factors, and treatment.' *Can J Psychiatry*. 2014; 59(9): 460–67. https://www.ncbi.nlm.nih.gov/pmc/articles/PMC4168808/#:~:text=Epidemiologic%20samples%20have%20demonstrated%20that,1%20lifetime%20comorbid%20mental%20disorder.&text=Some%20of%20the%20most%20prevalent,dependence%2C%20and%20another%20anxiety%20disorder.

[336] Stojanovich L1, Marisavljevich D. *Autoimmun Rev*. 2008 Jan; 7(3): 209–13. doi: 10.1016/j.autrev.2007.11.007. Epub 2007 Nov 29. PMID: 18190880.

[337] 'Posttraumatic Stress.' *Good Therapy*. https://www.goodtherapy.org/learn-about-therapy/issues/ptsd.

[338] Sareen J. 'Posttraumatic stress disorder in adults.' 460–67.

[339] 'Mental Illness.' Mayo Clinic. https://www.mayoclinic.org/diseases-conditions/mental-illness/symptoms-causes/syc-20374968.

[340] John W Barnhill, 'Overview of Trauma- and Stressor-Related Disorders.' *Merck Manuals*. (Apr 2020). https://www.merckmanuals.com/professional/psychiatric-disorders/anxiety-and-stressor-related-disorders/overview-of-trauma-and-stressor-related-disorders.

[341] 'Personality disorders.' Cleveland Clinic. https://my.clevelandclinic.org/health/diseases/9636-personality-disorders-overview#:~:text=It%20is%20estimated%20that%2010,above%20the%20age%20of%2018.

[342] Elea Carey. Timothy Legg, Ph.D. 'Psychosis.' *Healthline*. https://www.healthline.com/health/psychosis.

[343] S.M. Dillman, Psy.D. 'Common Therapy Approaches to Help

You Heal from Trauma.' *Good Therapy.* Mar 9, 2011. https://www.goodtherapy.org/blog/common-therapy-approaches-to-help-you-heal-from-trauma.

[344] Black, David S., et. al, 'Mindfulness meditation and the immune system: a systematic review of randomized controlled trials.' *Ann N Y Acad Sci.* Jun 2016; 1373(1): 13–24. doi: 10.1111/nyas.12998.

[345] Toussaint, Loren, et. al, 'Effects of lifetime stress exposure on mental and physical health in young adulthood: How stress degrades and forgiveness protects health.' *J Health Psychol.* Jun 2016; 21(6): 1004–14. doi: 10.1177/1359105314544132.

[346] Bruce Lipton, The Biology of Belief: Unleashing the Power of Consciousness, 10th Anniv. ed. (Hay, 2016).

[347] 'Difference Between MFT & LCSW Degrees.' Careers in Psychology. Pepperdine University. https://careersinpsychology.org/difference-between-mft-lcsw-degrees/#:~:text=Degree%20Standing,a%20master's%20in%20social%20work.&text=An%20MFT%20may%20possess%20a,in%20marriage%20and%20family%20therapy.

[348] 'LCSW vs. Psychologist.' Human Services Guide. https://www.humanservicesedu.org/lcswvspsychologist.html#context/api/listings/prefilter.

[349] 'Psychiatric-Mental Health Nurses.' About APNA. American Psychiatric Nurses Association. https://www.apna.org/i4a/pages/index.cfm?pageid=3292#:~:text=According%20to%20ANCC%2C%20the%20requirements,of%20continuing%20education%20in%20psychiatric%2D.

[350] 'Difference Between MFT & LCSW Degrees.'

[351] 'Memories of Childhood Abuse.' American Psychological Association. https://www.apa.org/topics/trauma/memories.

[352] Ralph Ryback M.D. 'Psychiatrist vs. Psychologist.' *Psychology Today.* Jan 24, 2016. https://www.psychologytoday.com/us/blog/the-truisms-wellness/201601/psychiatrist-vs-psychologist.

[353] Susanne M. Dillmann, PsyD. 'Common Therapy Approaches to Help You Heal from Trauma.' *Healthline.* Mar 9, 2011. https://www.goodtherapy.org/blog/common-therapy-approaches-to-help-you-heal-from-trauma.

[354] Bonnie Bright, PhD. 'Trauma and the Soul: Psychoanalytic Approaches to the Inner World An Interview with Jungian Analyst Donald Kalsched.' *Pacifica Post.* Pacifica Graduate Institute. May

23, 2017. https://www.pacificapost.com/trauma-and-the-soul-psy-choanalytic-approaches-to-the-inner-world.

[355] 'Common Responses to Trauma and Coping Strategies.' Resources. Trauma Center. http://www.traumacenter.org/resources/tc_resources.php.

[356] Haahr, Sven. 'Multiple sclerosis is linked to Epstein-Barr virus infection.' *Reviews in Medical Virology* 16 (5). https://doi.org/10.1002/rmv.503.

[357] Li S, Yu Y, Yue Y, Zhang Z, Su K. 'Microbial Infection and Rheumatoid Arthritis.' *J Clin Cell Immunol*. 2013; 4(6): 174. doi:10.4172/2155-9899.1000174.

[358] Rees, JH, et al. 'Campylobacter jejuni Infection and Guillain–Barré Syndrome.' *N Engl J Med*. 1995; 333: 1374–79. DOI: 10.1056/NEJM199511233332102.

[359] Swedo SE, Leonard HL, Garvey M, Mittleman B, Allen AJ, Perlmutter S, Lougee L, Dow S, Zamkoff J, Dubbert BK. 'Pediatric autoimmune neuropsychiatric disorders associated with streptococcal infections: clinical description of the first 50 cases.' *Am J Psychiatry*. Feb 1998; 155(2): 264–71. doi: 10.1176/ajp.155.2.264. Erratum in: *Am J Psychiatry*. Apr 1998; 155(4): 578. PMID: 9464208.

[360] 'Pediatric acute-onset neuropsychiatric syndrome.' National Institutes of Health. https://rarediseases.info.nih.gov/diseases/13087/pediatric-acute-onset-neuropsychiatric-syndrome.

[361] Ramey, S. The Lady's Handbook of her Mysterious Illness (Penguin, 2020).

[362] Feldman, Bonnie. 'An Invisible Epidemic. When your body attacks itself. Autoimmune Disease.' Jan 29, 2016. https://tincture.io/an-invisible-epidemic-when-your-body-attacks-itself-autoimmune-disease-5738b699de12

[363] Ibid.

[364] Ibid.

About Dr. Gary Kaplan

Gary Kaplan, DO, is the founder and medical director of the Kaplan Center for Integrative Medicine, and author of Total Recovery: A Revolutionary New Approach to Breaking the Cycle of Pain and Depression (Rodale, 2014). A pioneer and leader in the field of integrative medicine, Dr. Kaplan is one of only 19 physicians in the country to be board-certified in both Family Medicine and Pain Medicine.

He is board-certified in Medical Acupuncture and has studied and practiced Osteopathic Manipulative Medicine, Emergency Medicine and Herbal Medicine. In response to growing numbers of patients presenting with heavy metal toxicity, Dr. Kaplan received certification in the science and practice of chelation therapy, by The American College for Advancement in Medicine (ACAM).

In 1985, Dr. Kaplan created The Kaplan Center to offer patients suffering with chronic pain and illness a more effective model of medical care. Utilizing a broad range of conventional and alternative medicine strategies, the Center's physicians, nurses, psychotherapist, dietitian and physical therapists collaborate closely on patients' progress, sharing their insights and treatment recommendations to ensure the best outcome for each patient. This coordinated, multidisciplinary approach has proved to be highly effective — especially for patients suffering with complex and longstanding medical problems.

"My commitment is to take the time to listen carefully to patients so I can understand how and when the pain problem started, what treatments have been tried, and what has and hasn't worked in the past. My approach is offer to each patient their own individualized treatment program, integrating, as appropriate, both conventional and alternative medical approaches. My goal is to provide evidence-based medical care that supports and enhances each patient's natural ability to heal." – Dr. Gary Kaplan.

A clinical associate professor in the Department of Community and Family Medicine at Georgetown University School of Medicine, Dr. Kaplan was one of the directors of a $1.7 million NIH grant that funded an educational initiative to incorporate complementary, alternative, and integrative medicine into Georgetown's medical curriculum.

Dr. Kaplan worked with the National Institutes of Health (NIH) to establish acupuncture as a medically effective treatment for a range of chronic pain problems. Additionally, Dr. Kaplan has trained physicians in medical acupuncture through the Helms Institute for Medical Acupuncture, sponsored by the UCLA School of Medicine. A past president of both the Medical Acupuncture Research Foundation and the Virginia Osteopathic Medical Association, Dr. Kaplan has written and lectured extensively on acupuncture and the integration of complementary and alternative therapies in the treatment of pain and chronic illness.

In 2013, Dr. Kaplan was appointed by U.S. Secretary of Health and Human Services (HHS), Kathleen Sebelius, to the Chronic Fatigue Syndrome Advisory Committee (CFSAC). The Committee provides advice and recommendations to the Secretary of HHS through the Assistant Secretary for Health on issues related to myalgic encephalomyelitis and chronic fatigue syndrome (ME/CFS), such as access and quality of care for persons with CFS, the science and definition of CFS, and broader public health, clinical, research and educational issues related to CFS. Dr. Kaplan is one of four individuals on the 11-person Committee who brings special expertise in healthcare delivery, insurance, and the problems experienced by individuals with CFS.

In 2015, Dr. Kaplan established the Foundation for Total Recovery in order to provide support and find a cure for all who suffer with chronic pain and depression by educating patients, building an online community of patients, doctors and researchers, partnering with leading researchers, academics and innovators, and studying data to find a baseline approach to diagnosing and curing neuroinflammation.

The Kaplan Center = A More Effective Model of Care

Incorporating the best elements of conventional and alternative medicine, Dr. Kaplan's goal was — and continues to be — to provide an integrative approach that attends not only to a patient's physical symptoms but also addresses the root causes of an individual's pain and illness, including problems of the mind and spirit that may be contributing to the disease process. At the Kaplan Center, you'll find professional expertise, strong communication between you and your provider, and a high level of collaboration among the members of our medical team in caring for you. The result: We put you back in charge of your life and help you attain optimal health

Expertise

Our physicians are board-certified in medical specialties crucial to the non-surgical treatment of chronic pain and illness: family medicine, pain medicine, internal medicine, and/or medical acupuncture. Our medical team also includes licensed physical therapists, an acupuncturist, a psychotherapist, a nutritionist, a meditation instructor, a nurse practitioner and two registered nurses.

Communication

We partner with you by taking whatever time is needed to understand your symptoms, the onset of your condition, the nature of your pain sensations, and the therapies that have and haven't worked for you in the past. This gives our doctors the critically important time they need to delve into problem areas that otherwise might be overlooked.

Collaboration

We work as a highly coordinated, tightly integrated healthcare team. Depending upon your unique medical needs, your treatment plan may involve supplemental care such as physical therapy, nutritional counseling or stress management classes. On a regular basis, your case is jointly reviewed by all of the Kaplan Center providers you see to ensure that your care is carefully coordinated.

In addition, the Center's entire medical team, led by the Medical Director, Dr. Gary Kaplan, meets bi-weekly to discuss patient cases. This allows for the full range of the Center's medical expertise to be brought to bear on your case.

Results

You receive a more accurate, comprehensive medical diagnosis, an effective, individualized treatment plan — in writing and in plain English — and continual monitoring to evaluate your progress. In sum, we combine excellent medicine with a highly personal, time-intensive and integrative approach. This allows us to find solutions for chronic pain and other longstanding illnesses that have previously eluded effective treatment. Our goal is to return you to optimal health, and we won't give up on you.

This focused professional training, our uniquely integrative, non-surgical treatment approach, and our years of experience make us true specialists in successfully treating chronic pain and illness.

We are here for you, and we want to help. Our goal is to return you to optimal health as soon as possible. To schedule an appointment please call:
703-532-4892 x2

Made in the USA
Monee, IL
27 August 2023

41738100R00203